A Loving Weaning

How to Move Forward Together

WINEMA WILSON LANOUE

Praeclarus Press, LLC

www.PraeclarusPress.com

Praeclarus Press, LLC
2504 Sweetgum Lane
Amarillo, Texas 79124 USA
806-367-9950
www.PraeclarusPress.com

DISCLAIMER

The information contained in this publication is advisory only and is not intended to replace sound clinical judgment or individualized patient care. The author disclaims all warranties, whether expressed or implied, including any warranty as the quality, accuracy, safety, or suitability of this information for any particular purpose.

ISBN: 978-1-946665-03-4
©2017 Winema Wilson Lanoue. All rights reserved.

Cover Design: Ken Tackett
Developmental Editing: Kathleen Kendall-Tackett
Copy Editing: Chris Tackett
Layout & Design: Nelly Murariu

CONTENTS

Acknowledgements

My heartfelt thanks to the following people:

- Eric, for unwavering belief in me, for true partnership and love, and for being so stinking funny.
- My kids, for helping me become who I was meant to be and for teaching me how to truly love.
- My father, Dr. Mark Wilson, for lots of help with this project and for being a great example and a great Dad.
- My mother, Dindy Wilson, for showing me how to be a supportive, loving mom and for nursing all of us at a time when not many moms did.
- Leilani, for letting me bounce things off her, daily, for her excellent ideas and sense of humor, and for always being there
- La Leche League Leaders, past and present: Evalin, Laura, Jenny, Amy, Janine, Kat, Carrie, Julie, Susan, April, for being great examples and amazing women and friends.
- Lauren, Robin, Tammie, Allison, Laura, Cyndi, Reva and CeCe, for kind support and friendship throughout this process.
- Sally Butler Provo, for taking lovely pictures of me and for great conversation.
- Lydia and Savannah, for being such wonderful friends to my little one, when I was off working hard.
- Kathleen Kendall-Tackett and all the fine people at Praeclarus Press for such a valuable partnership and for helping me bring this book to fruition.
- the good folks at Next Door Bake Shop, Bollos, and Lucie Monroe's, for letting me sip and work and write most of this book in their establishments.
- All of the moms and babies I have had the honor of working with, for providing loving examples to the world and the inspiration for this book.

Weaning: A Unique Experience

I hope that you enjoy breastfeeding. I hope that you and your child have gotten to know each other deeply through nursing, and that your confidence as a mother is strong because of it. If you are reading this book, it is probably because you want to understand the weaning process, and want it to be a positive transition for your family. I applaud you for seeking information and for making loving choices.

As someone who works regularly with breastfeeding mothers and children, I like to define the process of weaning in this way: weaning is the unique experience you and your child have as he or she moves beyond the need to nurse for food, health, and comfort. Weaning *begins* when your child takes the first taste of solid food, and ends when your child no longer nurses. It is a process rather than just a product: a voyage rather than a destination. Your voyage will be completely unique because you and your child are unique.

What will make your unique experience a *loving* one? A loving weaning is one in which a child's self and needs are respected, as are those of parents. A loving weaning considers all emotions okay, and allows expression of them. A loving weaning is a shared experience that belongs to both you and your child equally. It isn't something either of you can do alone; it is a true partnership in which you move forward together.

For most mothers, the act of nursing, sometimes a hard-won victory, has been all about connection, and the deep relationship it has helped forge. The very idea of weaning can be a daunting one, a mysterious process that brings up feelings of fear and confusion. It may help you to know that this connection will not end as you wean. Your love has provided strong, deep roots that will support this relationship as it grows and changes.

Weaning may be your first opportunity to gently guide your child through a truly significant transition. You will need good information, compassion, and support for it to be what you want it to be. My goal in writing this book is to provide you with those things. After reading it, I hope you feel prepared and confident in your weaning journey and in your instincts as a mother. I hope that the process will bring you and your child even closer as you grow and learn together, in love.

Author Notes

Throughout this book, I present the experiences of parents to illustrate topics discussed, some of which were given to me for this purpose, and others that are amalgamations of many stories I have heard over the years. When these amalgamations are used, any similarity to a specific family or set of circumstances is unintentional.

Experts in gentle parenting and breastfeeding tend to use the same small body of language in regard to many of the topics this book covers. When I have been able to find the person from whom a certain term or phrase has originated, I have given them credit. Otherwise, I have considered them to be in common use.

I switch between genders when discussing children in this book, so as not to have to use the phrase "he or she" repetitively. Again, any similarity to anyone or any circumstances is unintended. Additionally, I want to acknowledge that there are people, both child and adult, for whom neither he nor she is appropriate and that there are breast/chestfeeding parents who are not mothers or who do not prefer the term breastfeeding, for whatever reason. I don't feel that I have the knowledge, at present, to be able to write well with this in mind, but I hope to do so in the future.

I use the word "weaning" for the entire process of moving past breastfeeding because I am writing in the United States; in other countries, "weaning" may be used to refer simply to the introduction of complementary foods to babies.

In this book, I often mention La Leche League International and Breast-feeding USA as available breastfeeding support groups because these are the most established, widespread, and familiar to me. However, there are many up-and-coming organizations that serve the same purposes and are providing great support. I encourage you to check out mom2momglobal (military) and Baby café.

What You Need to Know About Weaning

CHAPTER 1

Recommendations from Experts

Whatever your personal thoughts on weaning, it is always good to be informed as to the generally accepted professional recommendations, and to understand why they are what they are. Of course, there are many philosophies and recommendations out there, but I offer those of the American Academy of Pediatrics, the World Health Organization, and the American Academy of Family Practitioners because these are well-known organizations whose recommendations are based on good information and research about breastfeeding, as well as the needs of developing children.

Recommended Duration of Breastfeeding

There are many philosophies and recommendations out there regarding duration of breastfeeding. The American Academy of Pediatrics updates its recommendation regarding breastfeeding, which includes breastfeeding duration, every few years. It currently reads,

> The American Academy of Pediatrics reaffirms its recommendation of exclusive breastfeeding for about 6 months, followed by continued breastfeeding as complementary foods are introduced, with continuation of breastfeeding for 1 year or longer as mutually desired by mother and infant (Eidelman & Schandler, 2012).

The World Health Organization says,

> As a global public health recommendation, infants should be
> exclusively breastfed for the first 6 months of life to achieve
> optimal growth, development, and health ...Thereafter, to
> meet their evolving nutritional requirements, infants should
> receive nutritionally adequate and safe complementary foods
> while breastfeeding continues for up to 2 years of age or
> beyond (World Health Organization [WHO], 2017).

The American Academy of Family Practitioners recommends,

> Almost all babies should be breastfed, or receive human milk
> exclusively, for approximately 6 months. Breastfeeding with
> appropriate complementary foods, including iron-rich foods,
> should continue through at least the first year. Health outcomes
> for mothers and babies are best when breastfeeding continues
> for at least 2 years. Breastfeeding should continue as long as
> mutually desired by mother and child (Montgomery et al.,
> 2014).

Trends in childcare come and go, yet the recommendations of these and
other expert organizations regarding breastfeeding duration have been
reaffirmed, with very little change, time and time again. But you may wonder
why the recommendations are what they are. Noted pediatrician, author,
and gentle-parenting expert, Dr. William Sears says,

> We urge mothers to think in terms of years, not months, when
> contemplating how long to nurse. Breastfeeding is a long-term
> investment in your child. You want to give your baby the best
> emotional, physical, and mental start. Extended breastfeeding
> is nature's way of filling your baby's need for intimacy and
> appropriate dependency on other people. If these needs are met
> early on, your child will grow up to be a sensitive and
> independent adult. ... A baby's sucking need lessens sometime
> between 9 months and 3 years. The age at which this need
> lessens is individual, yet very few babies are emotionally filled
> and ready to wean before a year. Have confidence in your

intuition. While this beautiful breastfeeding relationship may seem like it will never end, you are laying a solid foundation for the person your child will later become (Sears, n.d.).

If you are interested in anthropological, biological, and cross-cultural aspects of human lactation and duration, you might consider the book, *Breastfeeding: Biocultural Perspectives* by Patricia Stuart-Macadam and Katherine Dettwyler. It offers an objective perspective and can also be helpful reading for partners and others, especially if they enjoy a more scientific view.

The Spectrum of Weaning Methods

There are many ways to wean, some of which are based on good breastfeeding information and gentle parenting practices, and some of which are not. What all acknowledged experts agree on is that abrupt weaning is never ideal for mother or child, and that it is rarely necessary. There can be physical and emotional concerns associated with abrupt weaning, and an ideal weaning pace would allow time for both mother and child's bodies and emotions to adjust to what may be a huge change for everyone.

Other than recommendations to avoid abrupt weaning, experts usually leave the exact methods up to parents. There are some great books and websites that give tips and techniques for encouraging the process, but most breastfeeding experts do not offer a lot of detailed step-by-step directions. In my opinion, this is good practice because prescriptive weaning directions do not fit all children, and they don't take into account your unique child and relationship. Mothers who try them often feel like they are failing at what looked like a straightforward process.

Most experts use the terms "planned weaning" (parent-led, scheduled), or "natural weaning" (child-led, unscheduled), when describing methods. In my observation, these are the extremes of what is really more of a spectrum, with "Completely Parent-led" on one end, and "Completely Child-led" on the other. In reality, the majority of individual weaning methods actually fall somewhere in between in response to the needs of everyone involved.

Parent-Led Weaning

As you would expect, weaning on the parent-led end of the spectrum occurs when the parent, or parents, take specific action to move the weaning process along according to an external time-table, with a specific age/end date desired. There may or may not be signs that the child is ready for this.

Parents whose weanings are mostly parent-driven can provide a compassionate transition by making sure that their plans are developmentally appropriate and kindly done. If parents are planning a weaning that occurs *before* recommended duration and signs of readiness, they will want to be particularly sensitive, and make sure that their plans are compassionately implemented, as babies are more at risk for health and emotional complications when weaning than older children.

Child-Led Weaning

A completely child-led weaning, in which a child nurses until he naturally moves beyond this developmental need and weans himself (often very gradually), is an unfamiliar idea for many parents in the U.S. In fact, the very name might sound as though parents themselves would have no say in the matter. "Child-led" simply refers to the needs and development of the child dictating the timeline, not to him making decisions that would override his parents' wishes.

Child-led weaning most commonly happens after 2 years of age, and it usually tapers rather than being an abrupt change. If your child seems to be abruptly weaning himself, *especially* before 1 year of age, this may actually be a "nursing strike." (Please see Chapter 5 for more information.) This kind of weaning looks different for every family who chooses it. It may mean that there is no curtailing of nursing at all unless it comes from the child. For other families, there may be no obvious curtailing, but parents may take advantage of natural opportunities that arise, promoting activities in which their children nurse less, and decreasing nursing in a natural, stress-free way.

This approach to weaning may even include some conscious work on weaning during specific times ("partial weaning"), especially when developmentally appropriate, and happily agreed to by the child. Usually, specific end date goals are only present if the child agrees to them, which is often easier than many families expect.

Whatever your methods ultimately look like, it is good to know that you can create the weaning that you are looking for. The key is compassion and responsiveness to the needs of the child being weaned, as well as to yours. Outside of abrupt weaning, the process can take weeks, months, or years. This will be unique to each family, according to their own circumstances.

Communication About Weaning

Working in partnership with our children means that we are striving to be as open as possible about what is being planned, and what is changing in their lives, especially when their bodies and relationships are directly involved. Sometimes parents worry about this kind of communication, wondering if discussion or preparation will build fear in their child. They wonder if it is better to just "rip off the bandage" with no warning.

As our children grow into adults, we want them to have sovereignty over their bodies, and their hearts and lives. Believing in the sovereignty of their young lives, now, with our job being to lovingly guide them, while respecting their bodies and hearts, is the best way for us to help ensure that this happens. "Ripping off the bandage" may teach them that they must always be on guard against someone doing something to them without their permission.

Obviously, how engaged our children can be in any weaning discussions depends on their age and development. We may not be able to do more than actively observe a 6-to-12-month-old baby, considering their personality and needs, to "include" them in the dialogue. Older children may or may not be able to take an active part, but they certainly understand quite a bit, and can benefit from the topic being gradually and calmly introduced.

Successful communication about anything that could cause emotional reactions requires that we speak and listen with respect and love. This practice of mindful, kind interaction is equally as applicable with children as with adults, and has been written about and taught by many different people. If you'd like more in-depth understanding of how to do this than I could ever give you, I recommend checking out the books, *How to Talk So Kids Will Listen & Listen So Kids Will Talk* by Adele Faber and Elaine Mazlish (an "oldie but goodie"), and *Nonviolent Communication: A Language of Life* by Marshall B. Rosenberg.

The Gentle Introduction

Many parents find it helpful to begin the weaning discussion long before they are considering working on it. They might mention the concept of weaning, as the opportunity presents itself, as something that happens for every child, like growing taller or learning to read, not as something that they are asking their child to do right then. For example, a child might be playing with an older friend and is interested in all the amazing things that that friend can do. Without any motives beyond introduction, the parent might remark that, along with the other things that the older child can do, she "doesn't need to nurse anymore" (making sure that they are not attaching any shame to this—not saying, "if you are a big kid, you shouldn't need to nurse either"). There are no value judgements, no applying it to their child directly, just a mention, as though it is a part of life—because it is! This introduces the idea to a child that, at some point, he will no longer need to nurse, and it does it in a way that doesn't carry any pressure with it.

Sometimes, when the idea of weaning is gently introduced, the child doesn't seem to react at all. However, he may have heard it quite well and just needs a chance to process it in a relaxed manner. Other kids may have a reaction, perhaps asking questions or getting worried. You can take that opportunity to just listen to how they feel and let them know that you will work together with them, when it is time, and that they will have a voice.

Further Discussion

When it is time for you to talk about weaning in more depth, whether you are allowing it to happen naturally, and just want to open communication or really want to step in and begin to plan, assess your emotional state before you start. Children can sense our emotions, and it is difficult to be at our best when we are angry, worried, or frustrated. You will want any discussion you have with your child to go as smoothly as possible, so if you are in the midst of negative emotions, take some time to breathe and work through them before you begin.

One proven way parents can practice compassionate communication is to truly focus on their children when talking, truly listening without judgement. You can assign innate goodness to your child and then try to understand her responses, without labeling any feeling as "good" or "bad." Sometimes the best thing to say is nothing. If a child has a strong response to the subject of weaning and says some version of, "I'm never weaning! I want nursies forever," it's okay to just listen, to give a hug, or to say, "I hear you. You love nursies!"

When you do this, it is easy to see that "I'm never weaning! I want nursies forever!" means that your child is afraid to lose the loving, treasured relationship that they share with you. You can accept that, and you can imagine how awful it would be to fear the loss of your mommy. You can assure her that you will always be there for her and that she will always be able to snuggle and be close to you (Rosenberg, 2003).

If you intend for your weaning to be at least somewhat child-led, you can simply continue to discuss weaning when it comes up naturally, avoiding pressure and answering questions and concerns. If you are planning to gently guide things a little more actively, you might begin to share your thinking with your child, and to ask them for their opinions. It doesn't matter if she says, "No." Many kids will say some version of "no" to new ideas. This is all about keeping that connection strong. Maybe you simply hug your child and say, "You love nursing, don't you?" Kisses, hugs, and nursing; if needed it; all of these tell her that it is okay for her to express her opinion and fears. Then, the next time you are in the store, you might go to the sippy cup aisle and let her look at all the cool designs, mentioning that she can use one of these if she ever wants to drink water during the night. No pressure. Over time, as it is gently discussed, she will become used to the idea.

If you are planning a more intentional weaning, on the parent-led side of the spectrum, you can still listen compassionately to your child's feelings, even if you don't feel that you can take as much time for him to get used to the idea. If you are cutting out nursing sessions and he has a strong reaction, you can tell him that it is okay to be sad (or mad or whatever). You can reassure him of your love and make sure he knows that this change does not mean that you won't be there for him. You can watch your own emotions and allow him to express his without any judgement (Faber & Mazlish, 2012). You can still find partnership and open communication in allowing him as much choice as possible in the situation. If you are planning to distract him during what used to be a morning nursing session, you can make sure to have a choice of distractions for him. If he is going to be held and rocked during the night instead of nursing, you can let him choose if he wants Mommy or Daddy to do it. There are still many ways for you and your child to communicate and be partners while weaning.

The crucial thing in any interactions between parents and children is not to get into a power struggle. There is no helpful outcome from a power struggle and, in fact, a lot of frustrating and unhealthy patterns can grow if you regularly get into them. As Mary Sheedy Kurcinka says in her wonderful book, *Kids, Parents, and Power Struggles,*

> If you win by simply outmuscling your child, you still feel lousy. There's little pleasure in victory when your child is left distressed

and angry. If you lose, it's even worse. What kind of parent can't even get a child to brush her teeth or finish her homework? ... Power struggles can leave you feeling scared and helpless ... Screaming at your kids wasn't part of your dream (Kurcinka, 2000, p.1).

If you need help avoiding power struggles and understanding how they happen, consider reading Kurcinka's book, or *How to Talk So Kids Will Listen and Listen So Kids Will Talk* by Adele Faber and Elaine Mazlish. Weaning usually happens early enough in your relationship that if you learn this now, you will get to feel the benefits of power-struggle-free communication for years!

CHAPTER 2

Your Child, Your Family, and You

Your individual breastfeeding situation and other personal considerations are just as important as professional recommendations. The success and ease of your weaning plans will depend quite a bit on your consideration of your child's personality and readiness. In the same vein, because no one is exactly like you, some methods will work for you and some won't, so your personality matters too (as well as that of others involved). Beyond that, your current home situation, family dynamics, and access to good supports play a part, so taking them into consideration as well will help you make a transition that works for everyone.

Personalities and Readiness

Is your child eager to try new things? Is he easily distracted, getting over hurt or frustration easily, allowing others besides you to help him? Does he need some control over situations, or is he happy to follow? Does he often choose play over nursing?

There never has and there never will be a human being exactly like your little one. No one knows your child like you do, and no one else can give his personality (which I like to think of as simply the particular way a person inherently feels and expresses their emotions and needs) the respect it deserves. Parents who accept, and even celebrate their children's personalities, find it much easier to create a unique weaning plan that really works.

Much of our ability to accept personality comes from our perspectives, and depends on whether we characterize personality and needs in a positive or negative light. A child who "wants attention all the time" might also be characterized as a loving and closely attached child who isn't yet ready to face the world without the safety of loving arms. That child is naturally very different from the child who runs off easily to try new things, and the only thing that will help her feel comfortable with more separation is if she feels safe and accepted until she is ready for it. This child may need the comfort of nursing, not just the food, in a more intense way than another child, and may need extra time, reassurance, and patience throughout the process.

In addition to your child's personality, his level of development and readiness for weaning must be considered because it may differ quite a bit from what is expected for his age, either by experts or by you. One child's emotional maturity at age 1 will look very different from another's. There are children who seem to understand quite a bit of what is going around them at a relatively early age, and may feel lots of confidence and excitement about trying new things that are meant for toddlers rather than babies. There are lots of kids who just aren't there yet. Developmental stages just can't be rushed. Keeping your specific child's readiness in mind, rather than just his age, will help you maintain realistic and kind expectations for him.

What About Your Personality?

Are you the type who can let something happen on its own, with no plan or timeline, or do you need a very specific strategy? Are you the kind of person who loves a lot of physical closeness and enjoys nursing an older child? Are you active and social, or do you need lots of quiet time?

Your personal feelings and intrinsic nature matter too, and paying attention to them provides a great example for your children, and helps them understand that you are unique, and deserve respect and consideration too. It also ensures that your weaning plan will reflect your feelings and nature, which will make it more likely to work well.

Family Situation and Dynamics

Your current situation and usual family dynamics matter too. Even if you are incredibly sensitive to your child's needs and your own, weaning can mean serious change, and trying to introduce even gentle beginning weaning techniques can be problematic if there are other stressful events happening, such as moving, divorce, a death in the family, a birth in the family, etc. At times like these, children need an especially stable and comforting environment that they understand and can count on, if possible. Asking them to drink a sippy cup of water during the night rather than nurse may be too much under the circumstances, and may actually set weaning back. Considering how much stress these situations can put on mothers, as well as children, initiating weaning may be too much for you too. Your energy, creativity, and ability to comfort your baby through the process may be compromised when, at another time, they it might be completely up to the job.

Family dynamics can be helpful to, or can hinder, the weaning process (and the breastfeeding process, in general). When extended family are closely involved, these dynamics can get even more complicated. If those close to a mother and child are clearly not supportive, or are openly hostile about breastfeeding, their expectations about weaning can impact mothers and babies. Children may not be able to comprehend everything that is said around them but they usually understand more than we think and, certainly, they absorb the climate and feelings of those around them, as Family Practitioner Dr. Katie Edson noted in a personal interview about weaning (personal communication, 2016). When children feel stress in the family, or perceive criticism or dislike of this thing that they love, they may cling more tightly to nursing rather than beginning to naturally move beyond it. Your weaning plans may need to include thoughts on how you will handle criticism. (Chapter 3 of this book has more discussion on this.)

Additionally, when mothers feel a lot of pressure from others, they may contemplate weaning long before they really want to. Moms often ask for information on how to wean but as the discussion progresses, however, they reveal that they don't feel ready to wean, but think that they must because of family pressure. In contrast, when the family dynamic supports breastfeeding, and mothers' choices are respected, they often feel able to explore ideas about weaning in a much more leisurely way.

If you are overwhelmed by family dynamics, please know that you are not alone, and that many women have been where you are. A mom-to-mom support group may help you with ideas to peacefully navigate your family dynamics. You may also need support from a professional counselor to be able to negotiate them.

Support

The support that you have, not only for breastfeeding, but also for your parenting, and for you as a person, can help make every phase of the breastfeeding relationship better, including weaning. As you consider weaning, assess your support system, and see if you need more help to wean in the way you truly want to.

Do you know other breastfeeding mothers who value gentle parenting, and who can talk with you about weaning? Getting good information and support about how weaning happens straight from someone who treasures nursing and can answer your questions can really bolster your confidence. Many moms find this information and support in a mom-to-mom group, such as Breastfeeding USA or La Leche League.

Do you have support for meeting your own needs? Often, moms turn to weaning when they feel that their own needs aren't being met. They wonder if this may be because they are constantly "feeding someone else's need." However, when moms are able to express their needs, and to meet them in some valuable way, such as spending time with friends, or having a chance to recharge or reconnect with their own interests, they often find that they don't feel the same frustration with nursing or other parts of parenting.

Whatever your personal breastfeeding situation, when you consider all of the important factors at play, you will better understand the weaning path that will work best for your family. Section Three of this book, "Making Plans," will help you figure out how these personal considerations can lead to an effective weaning plan.

Unexpected and Serious Circumstances: Discussion and Considerations

There are times when weaning just cannot look like our ideal of it; when life just takes over, and seems like it is making our decisions for us. The good news is that parents can be compassionate, even in challenging circumstances. Most situations do not actually necessitate weaning, despite what parents are often told. I have included discussions of several unexpected circumstances in the following pages so that you can feel informed and empowered to make your own decisions.

Mom's Illness or Surgery

Parenting while dealing with serious illness can be difficult to navigate and you may wonder whether your breastfeeding relationship can continue.

Here are some things to consider:

Who/what is telling you that you need to wean?

Have you researched your situation, or gotten more information from someone in the medical community who understands breastfeeding,

17

such as a Lactation Consultant (IBCLC)? It certainly makes sense that your health care providers might worry about your baby's exposure to medications via your milk, and if they would be liable if anything happened. As a result, they are extra careful, some of them recommending "pumping and dumping," or outright weaning all the time, as a precaution, no matter which drugs or procedures are being used with a nursing mother.

As always, it pays to talk to someone who has detailed breastfeeding knowledge and may have worked with moms who have used or undergone specific drugs and procedures. Luckily, finding information about breastfeeding and medications is so much easier now that Dr. Thomas W. Hale and Dr. Hilary E. Rowe have put out (and regularly update) the state-of-the-art reference book, *Medications and Mother's Milk*. Most breastfeeding counselors and Lactation Consultants have a copy, and would be happy to look medication information up for you, and many family doctors and pediatricians are now keeping copies on hand. You can also access this information online via the U.S. National Library of Medicine website, LactMed (toxnet.nlm.nih.gov/newtoxnet/lactmed. htm), a searchable database of information about medications and breastfeeding. You can also call someone at the Infant Risk Center (Directed by Dr. Hale, 806-352-2519), or visit their website (www. infantrisk.org).

If your questions relate to a procedure rather than a drug, or along with a drug, you can talk with a trained breastfeeding counselor (LLLI, BF USA, etc.), either locally or by telephone through their hotlines, or an IBCLC. Many times, they have worked with moms who have undergone the same procedure, and may even be able to connect you with them. You can also look online for information about your situation at Breastfeedingusa.org, LLLI.org (La Leche League International), and Kellymom.org (which is not a professional organization, but has many articles written by IBCLCs). You can also find support groups in person, and online, that may be able to help. LLLI.org and Breastfeeding USA have online directories for local groups and counselors, and

LLLI.org has a mom-to-mom forum on their website that addresses many breastfeeding/parenting-related subjects. This can be a great place to get help from Leaders and find other moms who know what you are going through. Additionally, Facebook now has pages and groups for all sorts of things, including moms who breastfeed in special situations, and these groups are very easy to access and join. As always, when online, or in any mother-to-mother discussion, just remember that you may hear things that are less than helpful. You may have to weed through suggested information to find what is correct and useful and medically safe. And, of course, make sure you are dialoging with your doctor as you proceed.

Being told to wean by someone other than a health care professional (a friend, a boss, a family member) can be even harder to deal with because you may have to see or talk to this person on a regular basis. But if you do your research, you can make your own decisions, and feel comfortable explaining them (or not), knowing you are well-informed.

What is your child's age and nursing pattern?

Drugs work in different ways. Understanding how the particular drug you need works, and how your child's age and nursing patterns come into play, may help you preserve nursing for a bit longer, if you wish to. Often, a drug that would be heavily contraindicated when nursing a small baby is not such a big deal when nursing a 2-year-old, and moms, in partnership with their doctors, are able to make a risk/benefit analysis of using it while nursing. Additionally, drugs have been classified into different safety levels, and take different lengths of time to process and leave the body. So, moms and doctors can work together to see if these drugs are relatively safe in the small amounts that might pass through milk, and to see if dosages can be scheduled so that they have mostly left the body before the next nursing session.

What if a drug (or procedure) has been proven unsafe for any amount of nursing?

There are almost always breastfeeding-friendly drug alternatives for most conditions, and even for some procedures, but your health care provider may not be aware of this fact. You may need to contact someone who has more information about these alternatives. The Infant Risk Center is a great resource for this information. Lactation consultants may be able to help you access information as well, and may have experience working with mothers in your situation.

If there truly is no possible alternative and you want to see what else you can do to continue nursing, you can consider whether a partial weaning would be safe. (See Chapter 10 for information on how to do this.) If your procedure or drug course will be relatively short, you can see if you can stock up on pumped milk to supplement with and return to breastfeeding as soon as it is safe. Additionally, if you know that you must wean to receive necessary treatment, you can ask your doctor if it would be safe to put off treatment for a short time so that the weaning can be a bit more gradual. If you have to abruptly wean, please see Chapter 10 for information on abrupt weaning.

Child's Illness or Surgery

When your child is very sick, the emotions and fear that you feel can be overwhelming. When health care providers tell you, in no uncertain terms, that you must wean, it can make things even more difficult. You know how nursing can comfort your child, and that your milk keeps her strong.

It is true that some parents find that nursing cannot continue while their child is being medically treated. With the right information and support, however, many find that it can, and that the nursing relationship helps keep some connection and normalization in what can be a very frightening process for both kids and parents. The important thing is for you to feel that you can make decisions from an informed place that takes into account both knowledge, and the needs of all involved.

If you are being told that you must wean, who is telling you so and why?

Again, health care providers will quite often make blanket statements about nursing to cover themselves legally (understandably). However, you may find, with further research and consultation, that breastfeeding can continue, though it may need to stop for a short period, or may need to change a bit.

For example, children often need to have an empty digestive system for surgery, and may need extended recovery time before taking any food by mouth. Many mothers have found that if they continued to pump regularly with a hospital-grade pump to keep up their supply, they were able to go back to nursing when their child was ready. Nursing was very comforting to both the mom and child. In other situations, moms have found that breastfeeding had to change a bit, such as when surgery required a long recovery for the child in which the child had to be tube fed. After discussion with doctors and Lactation Consultants, some moms have found that they could give their children pumped milk through the tube even though they could not nurse at the breast.

Whatever the situation, you will feel more confident in your decision if you talk with those knowledgeable about breastfeeding to see what your options are. Often, health care providers are more open than we expect to our wishes, especially if we can offer them good information to support them. Again, resources such as Lactation Consultants (IBCLC), La Leche League, Breastfeeding USA, and others can be very helpful in your research.

Difficulty Conceiving Another Child

There are many factors that play into the resumption of ovulation cycles and normal fertility after birth, and breastfeeding pattern is certainly one of them. This is the reason that the Lactational Amenorrhea Method (LAM) method of birth control has often been recommended to mothers, and has been found to be as successful as birth control pills (over 98 %) in preventing pregnancy when used correctly for the first 6 months after birth (Institute for Reproductive Health, 2017). Although some mothers will begin to menstruate and ovulate within the first 6 months postpartum, no matter how frequent and effective their baby's suckling is, most women's bodies begin to ready themselves for fertility sometime after those first 6 months. When, exactly, this will happen for you is still somewhat dependent upon your breastfeeding patterns, the unique nature of your body, and the unique nature of the sucking relationship you have with each of your children (they may all be quite different).

Mothers who are in constant physical proximity with their children, and who nurse frequently, including some "non-nutritive" sucking (nursing for sucking need/comfort, without taking in milk), with few long periods between nursing sessions, may find that their menses and/or fertility is kept at bay for quite some time. Breastfeeding mothers whose children go for long periods of time without nursing or who have replaced nursing sessions with solid foods at a young age may find that their menstrual cycles return quite quickly. And, of course, there are always those mothers whose bodies just do not follow any expected pattern as to breastfeeding and menses (Mohrbacher, 2010).

In most cases, mothers can conceive another child while breastfeeding, if their ovulation/menses cycle has resumed, though some mothers experience the return of menses long before the return of full fertility. Additionally, I have met some women who have not seen their cycles return, even though their children are over 2 years old, and they are no longer breastfeeding frequently at all.

When families have difficulty conceiving while breastfeeding, and look for help, they are often told that they must wean. While that is the case for a very small percentage of women, for most, a change in *how* they are breastfeeding can be very effective, and full weaning isn't necessary unless the family truly desires it. Many moms have found that by working with their child to postpone their early-morning nursing for a few hours, or by weaning from nighttime feedings, they have been able conceive without having to completely wean. Others find that shortening nursing sessions, spacing them out more, or replacing a few can help. Still, others find that a combination of these is needed.

Most mothers in the U.S. do not have a good understanding of how their fertility cycles work in general, or how breastfeeding and other factors can affect them. Books such as *Taking Charge of Your Fertility* by Toni Weschler, and *Your Fertility Signals* by Merryl Winstein can help.

Finding out how others have handled fertility concerns and nursing can be another way for you make well-informed decisions for your family. Mothers have found it useful to talk with breastfeeding counselors or other mothers, either in-person or online through breastfeeding-friendly forums, websites, and Facebook pages.

If you are one of those rare mothers who finds that they just cannot conceive while breastfeeding even a little, remember that you have given a wonderful gift to your child by loving him through nursing! Your needs and desires for your family are important, and there are ways to gently move toward weaning so that you can conceive. As always, an abrupt weaning is not indicated, as the stress and loss for both you and your child can impact your bodies and relationships. You can still complete your breastfeeding journey with compassion, and in partnership with your child.

Remember that there can be several possible reasons for difficulties in conception, and that weaning may not change an underlying problem. Be prepared to continue the process beyond weaning, should you choose to wean.

Difficult Working Circumstances

Working and nursing works for many mothers but some situations turn out to be very stressful. Active hostility towards the need to pump, store milk, and/or meet a child's other needs by a boss or co-workers can test any mother's dedication to breastfeeding.

It is wonderful that current law (as of this writing) in the United States requires that your workplace environment supports pumping (Murtagh & Moulton, 2011), but jobs vary widely in what they ask of a parent. Bosses and co-workers may be able to follow the letter of the law while still making you uncomfortable, so what the law allows may be the least of your worries.

It may be that, even with all possible preparation and discussion, your boss is pressuring you to be able to travel long before you are ready. Perhaps your co-workers openly resent your "extra breaks" for pumping, or you find that meetings last much longer than you expect, and clients can be offended when you need to leave. Perhaps you work in an industry where simply finding the right time to pump is challenging.

Trying to negotiate working and nursing without the support you need can be discouraging. Whatever the case, as always, you are the expert on what needs to happen. You will feel best if you are informed and empowered.

Here are some things to consider:

Is the pressure you feel to wean simply one more example of pressure that you often feel at your job?

Some bosses will push you to do more than you are comfortable with, no matter what your situation is. Like many women in our society, you may have been socialized to please others, and it may be very difficult for you to set boundaries and to stand up for yourself. It is important to consider whether the pressure you currently feel is truly just about breastfeeding, or if there has often been some sort of tug-of-war in your workplace, even before your child arrived. There may be skills in diplomacy and self-care that you will need to work on to make the situation better, whether you wean or not.

Some moms have reported that giving in and weaning because of work pressure made them feel like they had suddenly given permission for their boss or co-workers to criticize all other aspects of their personal lives, and that having to leave for a sick child became just as much a problem as pumping had been. They felt that they still had to learn the skills they needed to set appropriate boundaries, even after weaning. One mother I know stopped all explanations and apologies, and decided to only speak in simple "I statements." For example, "I cannot go on evening home evaluations until my daughter is at least 1 year old." She did this, and only this, and soon, no one asked her anymore.

Are you expecting weaning to solve your work problems?

Many moms say that they never feel fully invested in either home or work life while their children are young, and that they question continued breastfeeding because of this. I feel for them; it is a lot to ask of anyone to be able to be 100% committed to work and home life, both of which can require so much of you! It may seem like things would be completely different if you weren't pumping at work (and this is possible after your child is over a certain age – see Chapter 7 for more info). However, it is important to know that many of same work pressures and complaints are felt by women who haven't breastfed at all! Mothering small children *and* working a full-time job (or even part-time) can be difficult no matter what your choices are about feeding your child.

If you want to continue breastfeeding, and you want to keep the easy reconnection it provides you and your child, you may want to talk with someone for moral support and constructive ideas for making things easier. It can be nice to hear from other moms who have been in the same situation, and you can do this through groups like La Leche League (where working moms are increasingly common; in our local group, working moms are in the majority) and Breastfeeding USA. Additionally, there are Facebook groups specifically for breastfeeding and working mothers. If you are in the military, mom2momglobal is intended specifically for you and can be found at http://www.mom2momglobal. org/. You might also check out Robyn Roche Paull's book, *Breastfeeding in Combat Boots: A Survival Guide to Successful Breastfeeding While Serving in the Military*. Many mothers also find the books, *Nursing Mother, Working*

Mother by Gale Pryor and Kathleen Huggins, and *Working and Breastfeeding Made Simple* by Nancy Mohrbacher, to be very helpful in preparing for work and preventing difficulties.

Divorce and Separation

Separation and/or divorce while a child is small can be rough on everyone. There is often pressure to wean so that the other parent can have the child for extended periods and overnight. There can be milk-supply issues, as stress and separation take their toll. There can be nursing strikes and developmental regressions as babies and young children try to cope with emotional situations that they don't understand. There may even be pressures to wean because of custody battles in which the mother is portrayed as trying to keep the child from the other parent. Every family that works through divorce feels differently about breastfeeding and weaning, and there are no set rules or recommendations about this. It is up to you to decide whether weaning because of separation/divorce will help you, or make things harder for you.

Here are some things to consider:

How old is your child?

If your baby is quite young, especially if they are under 6 months of age, you can use the American Academy of Pediatrics recommendations to help others understand that your desire to feed your child only your milk, whether they are with you or with another parent, is legitimate and, considering that night-nursing is key for keeping up supply for most mothers, you may be able to explain that they need to continue to be with you at night, at least for the time being. If they are over this age, the statements of the AAP, WHO, and AAFP (listed in Chapter 1) may still be very helpful.

Do you feel clear about why you value breastfeeding, and comfortable explaining how important it is?

This list, put out by the Australian Breastfeeding Association (2013) is an excellent place to start. It says:

The precise nature of shared care arrangements will vary between families and may change over time. Nevertheless, the following points may assist families in working out the arrangements that work best for them and their breastfed child.

* Breastmilk is the normal food for babies, perfectly designed by nature for human infants.

* There are health risks for infants who are not breastfed, including increased risk of gastrointestinal infections, lower respiratory tract infections, otitis media, urinary tract infections, necrotizing enterocolitis, sudden infant death syndrome, and obesity.

* Breastfeeding must be exclusive to achieve the full benefit of its protective effects. Artificial feeding interferes with these protective effects:

  * Formula is an intervention with potentially negative health outcomes.

  * The first 6 to 8 weeks are critical in establishing breastfeeding. During this time, infants need unrestricted access to the breast to establish an adequate milk supply, and to develop the learned skill of breastfeeding.

  * Babies learn to breastfeed by breastfeeding—feeding them expressed milk (especially via a bottle) in the early weeks can cause significant difficulties in establishing and maintaining a successful breastfeeding relationship.

- Even after the first 6 weeks, the frequent use of bottles may lead to nipple confusion and/or breast refusal for some infants.

- Feeding a baby artificial milk has risks, for both the infant and the mother.

- Expressing breastmilk is not instinctive and is a skill that needs to be learned by the mother.

- The current recommendation is for infants to be exclusively breastfed until 6 months of age. This means an exclusively breastfed infant is entirely reliant on the mother for nutritional needs during this period.

- Breastmilk continues to be the most important dietary element in the baby's diet until 12 months of age.

- After 12 months, breastfeeding continues to be an important part of a child's experience, supporting their nutritional and emotional health.

- The World Health Organization recommends that breast-feeding continue for up to 2 years of age or beyond

(*Note*: The American Academy of Pediatrics recommends "… 1 year or longer as mutually desired by mother and infant.")

While most people understand that separation and loss can have a harmful effect on family mental health, few understand that breastfeeding promotes good mental health, and that parents can protect their children through this close physical connection. This kind of information can be very useful to all who are considering the needs of your child (Oddy et al., 2009).

How can you best meet your child's needs?

This time can be so difficult for children, whether or not they have the language to express their feelings, and whether or not they *seem* fine with the stress and changes in the family. Just like when moving, or making any major life changes, this may be a difficult time to add weaning stress on top of everything else, for your child and for you. Many moms find that, in the midst of upheaval, they just don't have the creativity and energy needed to find alternative ways to soothe and comfort their children. But it can be done. Mothers who decide to compassionately wean while under stress try to be particularly sensitive to their children's emotions, and consider ways to continue to lovingly meet their needs.

If your child will be away from you for significant amounts of time, pumping can help keep your supply up, and your child's other parent may be willing to give your milk rather than substitutes. Moms are often surprised at how willing others are to do this if they ask. It is good to remember that, in most cases, your child's other parent will want the best for your child, just as you do. Even when fed breastmilk by bottle or other methods, kids who are already established breastfeeders are often happy to nurse again when they are reunited with their moms. In fact, just as when mothers are working away from their children, this close, immediate reconnection can often set things back to normal more easily than anything else.

There are breastfeeding mothers who have gone through this before and, in my experience, they are eager to help. Seeking out experienced mothers for information and support may be one of the best things you can do.

Other Major Life Events

When there is a death in the family, a sick family member, or any other stressful life event that interrupts the peace of a breastfeeding family, fear and loss can be disabling, just as during divorce or separation. Often, getting through it as parents is difficult enough without the added pressure of helping our children through it. Yet, we must help them.

Just as in any other situation in which there is upheaval or loss, your ability to help your child through the added stress of weaning may be compromised and you may find that the easy reconnection that you find through breastfeeding is invaluable to all of you. Weaning, unless it is very gradual, can represent a loss for both mother and child, which may be more than some mothers can manage under the circumstances. Again, decisions about weaning and breastfeeding will center around who your child is, and what you feel you can handle. Remember that you can talk with other breastfeeding mothers about your situation, and that there are resources that can help you help your child, such as the excellent book, *Parenting Through Crisis: Helping Kids in Times of Loss, Grief and Change* by Barbara Coloroso.

In any difficult circumstances, if you worry that weaning may be necessary, but you'd really like to continue nursing, you might investigate whether a partial weaning could be helpful to you. (See Chapter 10 for more information.) Sometimes breastfeeding can survive a forced break. This can be the case when the special situation is surgery, illness, extended work travel, or mandatory time away from your child, such as military deployment or shared custody. It is true that some kids will choose to wean on their own if they take an extended break, depending on age and temperament. But many will happily begin nursing again as soon as they are able. Moms can keep up their supply during time away from nursing by pumping regularly, even if they cannot save this milk. The book, *Breastfeeding in Combat Boots: A Survival Guide to Successful Breastfeeding While Serving in the Military* by Robyn Roche-Paull, while intended for military mothers, is a great support for all mothers who experience long and short separations.

If all indications in your situation point to the need for weaning, and you are ready for that, consider how you will do it. Section Three of this book will introduce you to tips, techniques, and discussion of how to wean in a way that will best preserve your relationship with your child according to their age, readiness for weaning, and personality.

Frequently Asked Questions About Weaning

| # Negotiating Recommendations, Opinions, and Criticism

Q: Why do the AAP and others recommend at least a year of breastfeeding? Does this mean *just* a year or more than a year?

A: Epidemiological research shows that while any breastfeeding is better than none, there is a difference in health outcomes when a baby is breastfed for longer than 6 months, rather than stopping at that time. Incidence of gastrointestinal problems, ear infection, respiratory infection, and other sicknesses is lower in children who breastfeed for at least the minimum recommended time (Eidelman & Schandler, 2012.) While health is just one benefit of nursing until, or beyond the recommended time, this is the reason that the AAP provides in their statement, which is intended as a guideline for physicians to use as they advise and support mothers.

Children who are over a year old have more mature immune and gastrointestinal systems, are better able to understand the world around them, and may need the physical and emotional support of nursing a bit less than a younger baby. However, it isn't as though older babies suddenly reach maturity at one year and no longer need your milk or the benefits it provides. Your milk doesn't suddenly change from great to useless on your child's first birthday. It is a much more incremental process than that and, indeed, some benefits increase as your child grows, such as the density of immunological factors in your milk, packing a larger wallop into a smaller package, as older babies and toddlers nurse less, but encounter more germs than infants. Your body naturally provides for this and other age-specific needs (Newman & Kernerman, 2009).

This is the reason that the recommendation of the AAP is "for 1 year or *longer* as mutually desired by mother and infant" (italics added), and they are recommending that a year be the *minimum* length of time for breastfeeding. The World Health Organization and AAFP both advocate for 2 years or more and there is a vast amount of evidence on how this can benefit both mothers and children. What each family decides to do is completely up to them, but this is what is meant by the recommendation, and why it is the way that it is.

Q: How do I handle criticism if I wean differently than friends or family?

A: Your weaning will *always* look different from anyone else's. You and your child and your family are different than any other, and even if you were to follow someone else's program to the letter, there would still be differences. It is okay to embrace them! If and when someone feels the need to say something to you that feels critical, remember your expert status in your own family. You are the one who understands the needs and dynamics of your family, and you will be the best suited to decide how to handle parenting your child.

It would be lovely to feel a seal of approval from everyone around us, but it simply isn't possible. What is possible is to respond to criticism with compassion (often critical comments come from people who feel defensive about their own choices), confidence, and simplicity. "We're on the weaning journey and doing well" may be enough of an explanation, no details needed. If you are pressed for details? You might say, "We're following doctor's recommendations" (the AAFP and AAP are professional doctors' organizations so you *are* following doctors' recommendations if you follow theirs).

Most commonly, parents are criticized for weaning later than others think they should, but sometimes parents are weaning *earlier* than others would like. Again, confidence, compassion, and simplicity are key. It may be enough to say, "We are making the decisions we feel are right for us, and we respect your decisions too." Showing your continued loving connection to your child, and your attention to his needs, is the proof that this decision wasn't made lightly, or if it was forced upon you, that it was carried out with kindness and respect.

Q: My doctor told me I need to wean. How do I know if this is true?

A: Families are often told this but, unfortunately, at present, most health practitioners (except for IBCLCs) have not been well-educated about weaning. Your doctor may not realize there is rarely any reason that someone *needs* to wean, outside of some extraordinary situations (Montgomery et al., 2014).

If you are being told to wean you might consider talking in person to someone trained to discuss weaning with you, such as a La Leche League or Breastfeeding USA volunteer. You can also look at the previous section of this book on "Unexpected and Serious Circumstances," and the rest of these frequently asked questions in this section, many of which cover reasons moms are unnecessarily told to wean.

Q: My doctor recommends that I give rice cereal to my child at 4 months, but I just read the AAP recommendation that I should begin "about the middle of the first year." Several moms have told me that they are now introducing foods earlier to avoid allergies. What should I do?

A: Your baby's introduction to solid foods is his first step to weaning and, just like many aspects of parenting, how to do it can be confusing because of conflicting information and recommendations.

There has been a great deal of media hype surrounding a clinical trial that was carried out in the United Kingdom, and that many took to be evidence that solids should be introduced earlier than the recommended "middle of the first year." With some investigation, it turns out that only a certain group of at-risk babies were included in the trial, and the trial was specific to peanuts, not other foods. Yet, health care providers, and some mothers, have taken this as reason to begin offering many kinds of foods early for all babies (Fleischer et al., 2015).

As with anything, you can consider the doctors at the AAP *your* doctors, if that helps. At the time of writing this, they have not changed their recommendations that a baby be around 6 months of age when solid foods are first introduced (American Academy of Pediatrics, 2017). They may change this in the future, but until then, I tell moms that these doctors are tasked with critically reading all of the information that you and I can't, or wouldn't want to, and that if this information proves overwhelmingly game-changing, they will change the recommendations. Until then, they are telling you and your doctor what best practice is regarding infant and baby feeding.

If you think your doctor is open to you bringing up these recommendations, you may want to share them with him or her. If not, many moms find that it can be easiest to simply thank doctors for their suggestions and move on, realizing that they may have better information than their doctors do about breastfeeding babies.

Here is a great quote from La Leche League International's website (2016) on readiness for solids:

> Breastfed babies do not need to have complementary food introduced until about the middle of the first year. Before that time, you will notice some signs that your baby is changing

developmentally, in preparation for beginning solids in a few months. You will notice that:

- He becomes more sociable, playing and holding "conversations" with you during a nursing session.
- He has a growth spurt, and nurses more frequently for a while.
- He imitates the chewing motions you make whilst eating—he is practicing!
- You will know that he is *really* ready to start solids when:
- He is about 6 months old.
- He can sit up without any support.
- He continues to be hungry despite more frequent nursing that is unrelated to illness or teething.
- He has lost the tongue-thrusting reflex, and does not push solids out of his mouth.
- He can pick up things with his finger and thumb (pincer grasp).

Babies who are ready for solids can usually feed themselves. Mothers often report that they knew their babies were ready when they picked up food from a plate, chewed it, swallowed it, and wanted more.

Listen to your baby! Babies with a tendency to allergies may refuse solids until later in their first year. As long as they are growing well and are happy and healthy, there is no need for concern.

Q: I feel a lot of anxiety and pressure about weaning. Everyone says I need to "toughen up," and figure it out. Is it possible to wean without treating it like a battle I need to gear up for?

A: Absolutely! First, take a breath. It isn't a test or a battle. You aren't going to fail and, however you choose to do things, your child will wean.

Your journey can be one of peace. All children wean, and instead of it being a conflict, you can think of it as "getting where you were going anyway, but with a compassionate alliance." It is a bit like being on a plane that is going to make a safe landing. If it is going to get down on the ground no matter what, why not just read a magazine and let it land? Why pretend it is an emergency, grab a parachute, and jump out? Sure, you'll still get to the ground but, whew! Not the same trip.

It can really help to find mothers who have taken the gentler way before you, both for inspiration and for support. You can find them in person, and online in groups, like La Leche League and Breastfeeding USA. This may help alleviate some of your anxiety, and as you realize that you are already in preparation mode, just by learning about the process of weaning, you may feel less pressure.

Gentle parenting is widely recognized as important to the healthy development of kids, so your instincts are right on. Neither of you needs to "toughen up," and your loving way of life will be what truly makes weaning good.

Q: My partner and my parents are concerned I am nursing too long, and that my 10-month-old child is too dependent. They wish they could help more. Should I wean?

A: So many mothers ask, "how to wean" and, during further conversation, it becomes clear that someone else is pushing weaning, and that the mom and baby aren't necessarily ready. The question is: are *you* feeling ready to wean? This is something that primarily affects you and your child, and it is a process that you and your baby will want to feel good about, not pushed into.

There is so much misinformation passed around about breastfeeding, and people have very strong opinions that they are often too comfortable sharing. Pediatric experts all consider breastfeeding the best possible feeding choice that you can make, and experts also agree on the value of breastfeeding beyond the minimum requirements, and its role in fostering independence. Pediatrician, Jack Newman, and Lactation Consultant, Edith Kerneman (2009) say this about independence (and you could apply this to any extended breastfeeding, not just self-weaning):

> The child who breastfeeds until he weans himself (usually from 2 to 4 years), is usually *more* independent, and, perhaps, more importantly, *more secure* in his independence … Often, we push children to become "independent" too quickly … If a need is met, it goes away. If a need is unmet (such as the need to breastfeed and be close to his mother), it remains a need well into childhood, and even the teenage years … Of course, breastfeeding can, in some situations, be used to foster an *over*-dependent relationship. So can food or toilet training. The problem is not the breastfeeding. This is another issue.

Even when good information about the benefits of breastfeeding beyond a year is shared with others, it doesn't always stop them from pushing mothers to wean. Sometimes, it is necessary to set healthy boundaries with in-laws, extended family, and friends. Many parents simply say that they are following doctors' orders when questioned about weaning. Considering that the American Academy of Pediatrics recommends *at least* one year of breastfeeding, you *are* following doctors' orders if you do this.

If your partner and you disagree on how to proceed with nursing, it might be a good idea to consider talking with a licensed counselor about how to communicate with each other. The book, *Nonviolent Communication: A Language of Life* by Marshall B. Rosenberg, may also help.

CHAPTER 4 | Emotional and Physical Health of Mother or Child

Q: **I am pregnant. My toddler is still breastfeeding. Will this affect my pregnancy? What about when the baby is born and tandem nursing?**

A: Some women worry that breastfeeding while pregnant will cause miscarriage, or have some other negative effect. Sara Walters, writing for La Leche League USA's magazine, *New Beginnings* (2008), says that it is usually completely safe for a mom to continue to nurse her child while she is pregnant.

"However, if you are having a difficult pregnancy and are at risk for early labor, and in particular have been told to avoid sex during pregnancy, then weaning would probably be advisable."

Unless you are in this situation, the decision whether or not to continue nursing during pregnancy is up to you.

Of course, some moms who plan to continue find that nursing can become uncomfortable while pregnant, particularly if their breasts are sore or if they experience nursing aversion (strong negative physical/ psychological feelings when nursing). Some mothers find that their milk naturally dries up, or changes taste when they are pregnant (especially as colostrum begins to be produced), and their kids wean on their own because of this (though many don't). Other mothers nurse happily the whole way through pregnancy, and feel that it was an easy way to mother their older child at a time when they may have been tired, and less patient and creative than usual (Walters, 2008).

By the time your new baby is born, your milk will have changed to colostrum, and then will turn to "newborn milk" a few days later, even if you have continued to nurse your older child. Your body will provide everything your new baby needs because of the hormones of pregnancy and birth.

After birth, some mothers choose to "tandem nurse," which means that they continue to nurse their older child as well as their newborn, making sure that their newborn gets all the time at the breast that they need. While this may sound daunting, mothers who have done this often feel that their older child made the transition to older sibling more easily when able to share in the nursing relationship, feeling closer to the new baby, and less jealous than they might have otherwise. Some moms report that they felt more able to meet everyone's needs because of tandem nursing. Of course, tandem nursing isn't for everyone, but if you're interested in learning about it, the book *Adventures in Tandem Nursing: Breastfeeding During Pregnancy and Beyond* by Hilary Flower is a great place to start.

If you are thinking of weaning while pregnant, you should not find it any more difficult than at another time, save for your possible tiredness and your child's feelings about the coming baby. As always, you will need to provide compassionate support for him, with consideration for both of your needs. You should be able to use the same techniques as any other weaning mother.

Q: I have lost too much weight after my daughter's birth, and am having a lot of trouble gaining any. I feel like it isn't healthy, and I'm not sure if I am making good milk. Should I wean?

A: New moms often focus so much on losing weight, as a group, that the problem of losing too much weight can be overlooked and/or dismissed as "not a real problem." But it can be a real issue for some mothers!

Let me assure you that you are most likely making "good milk", just like anyone else. If your baby is growing and thriving, she is getting what she needs from you, and many moms in your situation have nursed to and beyond the recommended age. The question is whether *you* are getting what you need!

While making milk does require extra calories (the amount varies according to your body type and activity level), mothers don't usually need to wean to gain weight, but they may have to learn some new ways of eating in order to get enough calories for their own needs as well as their babies'.

Even though many nutrition experts have reversed their stances on fat, women in the United States still contend with the deeply ingrained idea that eating fat is bad for them. It is true that chemically altered fats, such as hydrogenated and partially hydrogenated fats, are damaging, but most natural fats are not. Indeed, fats are necessary for some functions in the body. Nursing mothers who are losing too much weight are often able to stabilize themselves if they add more healthy fats into their diets. Additionally, they may need to eat more often, which can be tricky with a baby! Over the years, I have seen mothers stabilize or gain weight with the following tips:

* Make a full blender of fat and protein-heavy smoothie in the morning, and drink some whenever you can throughout the day. Many moms report that adding coconut cream or full-fat yogurt is a delicious way to add fat to smoothies. Nut butters can be helpful in smoothies too.

* Keep a container of raw scrambled eggs, and one of cheese and/ or diced veggies or meat in the refrigerator, with a small, clean

pan ready on the stove, and some butter to cook the eggs in. Having everything ready means that eggs can be cooked quickly, and with one hand, if needed.

- Keep healthy-fat snacks on hand: avocados, olives, nuts, seeds, etc. Trail mix is great for a quick snack!

- Use whole milk, real ice-cream, full-fat sour cream, full-fat yogurt, real heavy cream, and whipping cream, etc. Stay away from anything that says, "low-fat" or "nonfat."

- Enjoy healthy oils in real salad-dressings, and in cooking (be careful to find out which oils are good to cook with, and which become unhealthy when they are heated).

- Keep liquids during meals minimal (unless they contain fat) to prevent false feelings of fullness.

- Eat snacks often. Keep them small (but nutrient-dense) enough to still feel hungry at meals. This may take some individual observation to regulate for yourself.

Remember that gaining weight won't happen overnight. If you can relax and allow for incremental changes, you will be able to make your weaning decisions based on what you want to do, and what your child is ready for, rather than out of worry for your health.

Q: I have postpartum depression, and I think nursing is contributing to it. Would weaning help with this?

A: I am so sorry to hear that you are going through this. Postpartum depression can be devastating to mothers, who hoped and expected a joyful transition into motherhood. I hope you know that feeling this way is not your fault and that many mothers have felt the way that you do. The admiration I feel for moms who manage to take care of their children under circumstances like these is boundless!

The causes of postpartum depression (PPD) are myriad and complicated, though research in the last decade has advanced our understanding a bit, so that we now know that there are: physical factors, such as pain, difficulty breastfeeding, sleep deprivation, stress responses, and personal chemistry and history; emotional factors, such as fear, sadness, and guilt; and psychosocial factors, such as distance from family or positive supports, strain with your partner after birth, and isolation.

While many mothers feel a mild form of short-term anxiety or depression after birth, it is not usually cause for immediate concern. They may be tired and stressed, but are still able to bond with their children, provide for their needs, and function (relatively) in their daily lives. The real concern is for mothers whose symptoms are serious and persistent and whose ability to function and enjoy life is severely affected. Experts say that this happens with a much higher percentage of mothers than you may realize, so you can be assured that you are not alone (Mohrbacher, 2010).

Mothers who contend with PPD experience real pain and doubt, and need help from the medical community and from their support systems. The breastfeeding mother diagnosed with PPD may feel further doubt and frustration if the support people they are looking to for help don't understand and respect the breastfeeding relationship. Often, it is especially helpful for these mothers to have other breastfeeding mothers to talk with. If you don't know any other nursing families that you can speak to (and who may also have breastfed with PPD), groups like La Leche League and Breastfeeding USA will be able to provide an opportunity to meet them and speaking with a trained breastfeeding counselor from groups such as these can be an important step for finding positive supports.

Some mothers who struggle with PPD feel that breastfeeding is helpful to them, emotionally, in that it encourages closeness and bonding, releases oxytocin into the body (the "love hormone"), and helps them get more sleep than if they were preparing and using bottles. Some of these mothers report that breastfeeding is the only time they feel like "good" mothers. Some feel that continued breastfeeding encourages them to interact with their children when they might otherwise be prone to isolate themselves.

Sometimes breastfeeding mothers feel that their PPD was triggered by problems with initiating or sustaining early breastfeeding. These problems, as well as traumatic birth, can take the form of a kind of posttraumatic stress. Hilary Jacobson, in her book, *Healing Breastfeeding Grief: How Mothers Feel and Heal When Breastfeeding Does Not Go as Hoped*, provides a valuable resource for working through this issue. I often recommend this book to mothers as a support for their journey, whether or not they are still breastfeeding. If this is the case for you, you may benefit from this book, as well as work with a licensed counselor.

There are other nursing mothers who experience PPD and feel as though *continued* breastfeeding is causing it or making it worse, perhaps because it remains difficult or painful, or because it is perceived as interfering with sleep or other parts of life. When breastfeeding is going well, it truly can be a light in the darkness. When it is not going well, when supply or latch issues persist and/or there is pain, moms can feel like it is standing in the way of their well-being. In these cases, solving the underlying cause of the discomfort, finding ways to get more sleep and promoting better mental health in other ways can help quite a bit.

When depressed nursing mothers see their health care providers (including counselors), they may find that the health care providers know about PPD, but don't understand the needs of the breastfeeding mother and baby. They may recommend weaning, out of hand, in a desire to immediately "fix" the problem, without understanding how breastfeeding works, and how it can actually be beneficial for mental health and for sleep. Anecdotes of mothers who experience PPD for the first time, or a worsening of their PPD symptoms after weaning, are so common in parenting circles that health care providers would do well to take more time to understand the individual situations of each mother before recommending weaning, especially as many medications that could be helpful are considered safe for nursing babies. Also, before recommending medications, or unnecessary weaning, your health care provider should rule out other conditions, as stated here.

> Clinical evaluation of postpartum symptoms must also include screening for thyroid disease, anemia, and diabetes, since these disorders can mimic symptoms of mood disorders (Slevin, 2007).

As you seek help, you might consider what role breastfeeding has been playing for you. You might ask yourself whether nursing, itself, has been difficult or painful, or whether you simply associate it with sleep deprivation, or yet another way in which you are not in control of your body: on-call to give of yourself no matter how you feel. Resentment is not a good motivator for anyone, and for some mothers who feel resentment *specifically* about breastfeeding, but not about the other parts of caring for their baby (including other methods of feeding), weaning may change things (though resentment can often be eased for many of these mothers through other means, as well). If, on the other hand, you find that you resent *most* parts of parenting and feel overwhelmed by most care activities, you may need interventions that are broader than weaning because your child will still need the same amount of care (and some would say more, because of the added duties of bottle washing, using other means to comfort, etc.).

If breastfeeding at night feels like it is contributing to the problem (and lack of sleep certainly can be a great stressor), you might ask the same questions. Is it the nursing itself that is the problem, or are you lying awake and restless after the baby has gone back to sleep? If you have insomnia, you will need a broader intervention than weaning (especially as your baby will still wake and need help during the night if you wean). Remember, too, that studies show that exclusively breastfeeding mothers who nurse at night actually get *more* sleep than non-breastfeeding mothers, though the general perception of this in our culture may be the opposite (Kendall-Tackett, 2017). Some tips for how parents of small children can get a little more sleep are in Chapter 5 of this book and may be helpful for you.

There are many interventions that mothers have found helpful in treating PPD. Some of these are pharmaceutical antidepressant medications and your doctor or Lactation Consultant should have access to Thomas Hale and Hilary Rowe's book, *Medications and Mother's Milk* so that they can check the safety of these, many of which are considered safe. If they do not have a copy they (or you) can speak to someone at the InfantRisk Center, founded by Dr. Hale, at (806) 352-2519. However, many mothers may consider medications a last resort and there are non-medication interventions that have been found to be very beneficial. Here are some of these:

* **Get help to resolve any current breastfeeding issues.**

International Board Certified Lactation Consultants (IBCLCs) are often quite willing to see mothers as their babies grow beyond the newborn stage and trained volunteers with groups such as La Leche League and Breastfeeding USA, provide their services for free to any mother who needs them. Figuring out what is behind pain or supply issues may help relieve a good deal of stress.

* **Assess your nutritional situation.**

Mothers who are low in important nutrients or important vitamins can be much more prone to depression and other conditions. While there are many important nutrients to consider for your general health and well-being, expert Kathleen Kendall-Tackett (2017) points to studies that show the vital importance of Omega-3 Fatty Acids in mental health and their use in combating depression.

* **Assess your sleep situation.**

Sleep is the one thing that makes or breaks it for some mothers. Sleep is incredibly important for good mental health. As previously discussed, when it comes to night-time parenting, reports indicate that formula-feeding mothers experience higher levels of exhaustion than breastfeeding mothers, overall, which is often at odds with the knee-jerk recommendation to wean that some health care providers have upon hearing depressed mothers are nursing during the night

Yet, even breastfeeding mothers can feel overwhelmed by baby's waking, or by insomnia. Some mothers get better sleep by moving the baby into bed with them, or by finding some other close sleep arrangement that allows for the least disturbance possible. There are ways to co-sleep safely and this and other helpful information for getting baby to sleep a bit better can be found in the book, *Sweet Sleep* by Diane Wiessinger, Diana West, Linda J. Smith, and Teresa Pitman, and *Gentle Sleep Book: For Calm Babies, Toddlers, and Preschoolers* by Sarah Ockwell-Smith.

Other mothers lower their expectations in other areas of life in favor of sleeping during the baby's naps, or find other creative ways to get a little more rest, if waking with the baby is the problem (See Chapter 5 of this book for ideas).

If mothers are up even when the baby is not, there are safe ways to try to help with this, including exercise, herbs, and supplements (always check a book like *The Nursing Mother's Herbal* by Sheila Humphrey or *Medications and Mother's Milk* by Thomas Hale and Hilary Rowe for safety with these), and psychotherapy which is specifically helpful because so many mothers are living with fear and/or past or present trauma that can make sleep difficult (Kendall-Tackett, 2017). And, as much as mothers may hate to hear it, some of us are just extremely sensitive to caffeine (and some of us find it affects our babies too), and find that our sleep is vastly improved when we kick the caffeine habit. Many moms also report that they feel *more* awake during the day when they are not using caffeine because they have no "crash" when it has worn off.

✸ Get more exercise.

It can seem hard to do this when you aren't feeling motivated, and when all of your time feels taken up with just getting through your day, but exercise is monumentally helpful, for the general symptoms of depression, and for sleep. Here are just a few ways that exercise helps with depression (among many): getting exercise produces endorphins and lowers inflammation (a stress-response cycle linked with depression) and exercising out in the sun can raise vitamin D and serotonin levels, all of which are great for mood. Walking, jogging, or hiking outside is free, doesn't require you to find childcare if you have a baby carrier or stroller, and can provide further mood elevation as you begin to feel good about doing something healthy in your life. In short, anything you do to be active can only help your mood (Kendall-Tackett, 2017).

✸ Eat as well as you can.

I know this is another difficult one when you are feeling terrible, but junk foods make us feel worse, not just physically, but also emotionally, because we can be overcome with guilt or worry when we do things that we know aren't good for us. "Comfort food," if it isn't healthy comfort food, can quickly make us feel worse than we felt before we ate it. This is an area where support can be key. You may not feel like you can handle the grocery store or cooking, but a partner or friend may be happy to help you get or prepare healthy snacks or meals for your day. Some moms find that just having fresh fruit or a bag of trail mix that they can dip into makes a big difference. Here is another area where a support group of moms may have lots of great ideas for you.

✸ Spend time with other moms, friends, family: whoever feeds your spirit.

Sometimes struggling moms don't like to be around moms at baby classes or the park because they feel worse seeing how these moms seem to be joyfully perfect in their motherhood. Similarly, old friends who expect certain things from you that you cannot give can be draining.

Seek out social interactions that elevate you. For many moms, this is found in mother-to-mother support groups, such as La Leche League or Breastfeeding USA, partly because mothers in these groups regularly share and comfort each other through the difficulties of parenting, rather than just keeping things on a superficial level.

If you don't have a mothering support group near you, or just prefer one-on-one social time, you might look for ways that you and your partner or a friend can go out and enjoy yourselves in the community, with or without having to spend much money or leave your baby. You may even be able to combine your social time with exercise, walking with a friend while your baby is in a baby carrier or stroller.

Whatever you do, most women need some sort of social supports to feel at their best and this can be so easy to neglect as new mothers. Effort in this area isn't wasted or selfish (Kendall-Tackett, 2017).

✸ Consider counseling.

There are many kinds of therapy, and many different therapists. It may take you a bit of time to find the right fit. Many people, moms included, have found great relief when talking and working with a good counselor or psychotherapist. Just being able to open up and get those "forbidden feelings" out to someone who doesn't have a stake in your life can be such a great release, and learning how to recognize and process emotions can help mothers heal and move forward. For many women who have experienced trauma, working with someone trained to help can be hugely beneficial, in every area of parenting and life. Just like exercise, personal therapy can be as effective as medical treatments (Kendall-Tackett, 2017)

- **Consider herbs and supplements and other therapies that can elevate mood without affecting the breastfeeding relationship.**

Herbs, such as St. John's wort (the most studied herb for depression), Omega-3 fatty acids (as discussed above), bright light therapy, and other non-drug treatments for depression can help with your symptoms. As always, make sure that they are safe for you while breastfeeding and that they do not affect milk supply by consulting a resource such as *Medications and Mother's Milk* by Hale and Rowe, or talking with your doctor. Make sure to check with your health care provider to make sure that anything new that you want to try will not interact negatively with other drugs or supplements you take. Many people forget to or feel uncomfortable telling doctors about what supplements they are taking, but it is very important to do so.

Note: Pharmaceutical antidepressants and St. John's Wort should not be used at the same time (Kendall-Tackett, 2017).

- **Be open with significant others in your life.**

Many mothers struggle with this. They don't want to let anyone down, or cause their partners to fear for them or their children's safety. They don't want to be judged or looked down on for not feeling euphoric about motherhood, or not being able to cope with what others seem to handle just fine. They may be hesitant to talk out loud about what is going on because they are afraid that they will break down completely. You may feel this way too. Just remember that no one can help you if they are fooled into thinking that you are happily "having it all."

Sometimes, moms think that they are clearly telling their partner or others that they are having a tough time, but they aren't actually getting their message across. Other people need you to clearly say what you feel, and what you need. Your reactions to what others say or do (tears, irritability, anger) may feel like communication, but they may not say anything helpful at all when translated in the other person's brain. What moms really want is understanding and help, so they need to be heard.

Sometimes, feelings must be simply spelled out:

> I am feeling depressed. I still take care of our baby, but I am
> not enjoying anything, and I think I need help. I am looking
> for ways to get better and I need you to help me by ...

It is always best to give ideas as to what you think would be helpful to you in as clear terms as you can (for example, just listening when I am feeling negative; taking over some food preparation for a while; taking the baby after I nurse her when I come home from work so I can have a few minutes of alone time, etc.).

Just getting those feelings out, just speaking them without the world ending or those around us judging us, can be a great relief. If you need help with this communication, a counselor can be helpful, and the book, *Nonviolent Communication* by Marshall B. Rosenberg, may also be helpful.

Whatever you end up choosing to do in regard to depression and breastfeeding, remember that you have already accomplished something wonderful for your child by nursing him, no matter how long you continue. You have already done more than many women are willing to do under the best of circumstances. We are all just trying to survive and thrive, and you deserve to find your way to joy in parenting just like anyone else. I am not an expert in PPD and I know that I cannot completely address a subject as complicated and individual as this, but I hope that you can come away with a little hope, both for yourself and for breastfeeding, if you choose to continue. If you, your partner, your counselor, or your doctor would like to read more about PPD and breastfeeding, the book, *Depression in New Mothers, 3rd Edition,* by Kathleen Kendall-Tackett is absolutely full of well-researched information about this subject and would be a valuable resource for anyone working with new mothers.

Q: **Lately, I feel like my supply has dropped, and my 7-month-old seems less interested in nursing, and just wants to be on the go. I can't feel a letdown anymore, and if I don't nurse for several hours, I don't feel full. Is it time to wean?**

A: Our bodies change a lot throughout our nursing journey. Moms are often concerned that these changes mean that they have less milk for their children when, in fact, it can mean that their bodies are finally making the right amount on demand.

Some moms worry about supply because of their children's behavior, which they believe signals dissatisfaction. There are many reasons for a baby or toddler's behavior to change, and most of them are not related to a change in your supply, though a baby may nurse more to encourage an increase when a growth spurt is coming, or has already begun.

These are signs of change that ***do not*** signal a lowered milk supply:

* **Breasts feeling less full and/or no leaking or feeling of letdown.**

This often happens when your body and your baby are finally perfectly in-sync. It can happen when your baby is a few months old, or quite a bit older. You are no longer producing more than your baby needs at times when your baby doesn't need it. You have truly become an "on demand" food source, and this is a positive thing.

Note: Some mothers *never* feel engorged, and *never* feel a letdown in their entire breastfeeding relationship!

* **Low or lowered pumping output (a "slump").**

Pumping output is not a very good indicator of how much milk a baby gets from the breast. In fact, women with very ample supplies often can pump only a few drops at a time in the early days of pumping. Mothers' bodies often must learn to respond to a pump, and some never do well with this, even though they have more than enough for their children. Additionally, some mothers who have pumped well in the beginning may find that their pumping outputs suddenly lower as their bodies and their children go through natural changes. This is not usually a sign of general supply difficulties (i.e., when your baby is at the breast), but may be a sign that your body is under a stress, or that your hormones are changing. Usually, a temporary extra daily pumping session or two, and massage during pumping, takes care of this.

✹ Child nursing very quickly.

Just as mothers' milk-making becomes more efficient, children's ability to take in that milk become more efficient. It is not uncommon for babies to get what they need in as little as 5 minutes so this, by itself, is not a cause for worry.

✹ Child fussy during or after feeding, and seems to want more.

There are so many reasons for a child to be fussy during or after nursing: teething, gas, onset of sickness, tiredness, overstimulation, ear infections, thrush, etc. Most of these issues resolve themselves naturally, often without us ever knowing what the cause was. Sometimes, when babies have eaten enough, but haven't completely satisfied their sucking needs, they can get frustrated and would be happy to suck on a clean pinky or a pacifier if they are old enough to take one without jeopardizing breastfeeding. Other times, babies have become so efficient that they are done, and the mom hasn't yet figured out this new nursing style, and tries to keep them on the breast.

✹ Child distracted while breastfeeding.

At about the middle of their first year, babies go through a major developmental leap, and get incredibly excited about everything around them. This certainly changes the nursing dynamic! But it is very normal and, thankfully, it doesn't last forever. It is about development and not about you or your milk. I promise that your baby still loves nursing and does not want to lose it. She is developing normally, and watching and learning at a ferocious pace. Sometimes, those distracted nursing sessions lead to a bit more nursing at night, just to get the calories in when there is less distraction, so be aware that that is normal too. Luckily, there are things that you can do to try to help the situation a bit. (See Chapter 5 for tips.)

✴ Child has fewer poopy diapers.

It is surprising how often people forget to tell a new family that exclusively breastfed babies typically begin to poop less often at around 6 weeks of age. They may go from reliably pooping several times a day to pooping once every few days, or even less. This is normal, as the gut matures, and is only concerning if the baby seems extremely uncomfortable (though a little discomfort when finally getting that large poop out is normal) and upset. This is not a sign of a lower milk supply unless, perhaps, it is coupled with other symptoms that the baby is not getting enough (such as not peeing often enough, losing weight, failing to thrive, etc.).

✴ Child wanting to nurse more often.

This is usually your baby's very effective method of telling your body that she needs more milk because she is about to have a growth or developmental spurt. It is really a lovely example of supply and demand working just as it should, and it typically doesn't last long.

✴ Child waking more at night.

This can also be due to your baby doing some good work on the demand side of supply and demand, especially as the hormones responsible for milk production can be higher in the wee hours. She knows what she is doing! It can also be due to other factors, such as distractibility while nursing during the day (making up for lost calories), developmental leaps, or teething (or other) pain. Whatever the cause, this extra wakefulness doesn't last forever, and you aren't hurting anything by nursing and meeting your child's needs during the night.

✳ Child's weight gain has slowed.

The rate at which a breastfed baby gains weight from one doctor's visit to the next does slow for many babies as they near the middle of their first year. This is normal, and unless the baby is losing weight (not just lower in percentile than they were), not gaining at all, or not peeing very much, it is not usually a reason to worry about your supply, though health care practitioners often prefer that babies maintain a continuous rate of growth even though that is rare (Mohrbacher & Kendall-Tackett, 2010).

So, what *are* possible signs that your supply could really be lower with your older baby? If your child's pee output has changed significantly (older children pee less often than newborns, but the amount is much more), and he is losing or not gaining weight, you may want to talk with your Lactation Consultant and/or doctor. Usually, the solution for lowered supply is nursing or pumping more for a while to signal to your body that an increase is needed, though some foods, herbs, and medications can be helpful. Supplementation may or may not be necessary and can make your supply problems worse if it isn't done correctly.

Q: Breastfeeding has not been easy for me—ever. I have always had pain and supply issues, no matter how much work I have done. I am very proud that I stuck with it for 11 months, and I want to quit as soon as my son is 12 months old. Is that okay?

A: I am always amazed by moms who nurse through such adversity. What incredible devotion and love you have for your child! After all you have been through, your instincts are sharply honed, and you really are the expert on what is right for you and your family. If you feel that you and your son are ready to begin weaning very soon, then you can feel confident about your decision.

If you think that you might feel differently if your issues were resolved, and you have already worked with a Lactation Consultant and others, you might contact a different International Board Certified Lactation

Consultant (IBCLC), La Leche League Leader, or Breastfeeding USA counselor. Sometimes, a new helper has that one bit of information that changes everything, and makes your remaining nursing time more enjoyable.

The important thing is to remember that a good weaning is often a slow process. That end date of 12 months does not mean that things will change that day, unless you are abruptly weaning, which can be uncomfortable and traumatic for both you and your son. But you can begin your planning now so that you are ready, knowing that every step you take is a step toward full weaning. Please see Chapters 8 and 9 in this book for information on how to make a weaning plan.

Q: My daughter already has cavities at 17 months old, and my dentist told me that it was because of nursing. She basically said that I need to stop nursing immediately, especially at night! Do I really need to wean?

A: There is a lot of misunderstanding about dental caries and breastfeeding. To further confuse the issue, some dentists make recommendations based on old case studies rather than on the newest and best information out there. Many dentists have had no education at all about breastfeeding, other than being told that *any* feeding at night will lead to "bottle mouth" cavities, though that information is based on children who bottle-fed, not breastfed, at night. Whatever the age of the child, breastfeeding itself has not been shown to cause cavities, though certainly breastfed children can get them (Iida et al., 2007; Mohebbi et al., 2008).

Cavities in baby teeth have several possible causes: bacteria (*Streptococcus mutens*, especially), genetics, maternal health during pregnancy, fetal development, oral hygiene, and diet, to name just a few. A breastfed child's decay usually isn't anyone's fault; the conditions for it most likely happened in utero and/or through contact that spread *S. mutens* from someone else's mouth to the baby's mouth (see more below), and the thing to do now is to keep those teeth as clean as possible, trying hard not to allow food, (other than breastmilk alone) to stay in the mouth, especially at night, feeding *S. mutens* and causing further decay.

Streptococcus mutens is a bacterium, colonies of which are present in the mouth of most adults, in differing amounts, and it is one of the primary causes of tooth decay, in part because of how it uses carbohydrates and lowers the PH level in the mouth, creating the perfect acidic environment in the mouth for decay, especially in vulnerable teeth (Forssten et al., 2010). Transmission of this bacteria is a major factor in childhood dental caries, whether babies are breastfed or not, and it can happen in any situation where the saliva of another person comes into contact with a baby's mouth–through sharing utensils or cups, through kisses, through food sharing, through babies thrusting their fingers in the mouths of others, etc. In other words, it happens very easily and the idea that mothers could keep this from happening by non-stop physical vigilance seems almost impossible, especially if the child plays with other children or is taken care of by other caregivers (Berkowitz, 2006).

Recent promising research leads many dentists to recommend that mothers chew xylitol gum several times per day to try to prevent initial transmission of S. mutens. These studies seem to show that xylitol greatly reduces the amount of *S. mutens* in the mother's mouth, lowering the incidence of transmission and colonization of the child's mouth. However, the American Academy of Pediatric Dentistry (AAPD) does not yet consider these studies to be conclusive and recommends that more studies need to be done before it officially recommends this. Additionally, some dentists are recommending xylitol as further decay control for babies and children themselves, in the form of paste and wipes, but this has yet to be recommended by the AAPD (who considers present studies to be inconclusive, as well) and the safe, effective amount for prevention in children has yet to be determined (American Academy of Pediatric Dentistry, 2015). While xylitol has been around for decades, the regular consumer use of it is relatively recent, and some families are concerned about its unknown impact on overall health long-term and its manufacturing/refining process, though it originally comes from a natural source. If you are interested in the use of xylitol, or other methods of prevention, do some research and speak to your dentist for a professional recommendation. *Note:* Xylitol can be fatal for dogs, so make sure to store it safely if you are using it in a household with dogs!

If your child has decay, then *S. mutens* is most likely already present in her mouth, though maternal use of xylitol may still be helpful. The good news is that breastmilk, alone and not in the presence of any other foods, *also* decreases *S. mutens* in the mouth, and diet and good oral hygiene can also be very beneficial, both for your baby and for you.

So, what happens when the breastfed baby nurses at night? Those who are familiar with breastfeeding mechanics knows that the nursing child pulls the nipple deeply in, and as the milk is extracted it is quickly swallowed. When this sucking at the breast stops, the milk stops, unlike sucking on a bottle, in which the milk can continue to come out even when sucking ends, pooling in the mouth or behind teeth.

If breastmilk, on its own, *were* to sit in the mouth, it still would not cause the same problems as formula because one of the many beneficial components of breastmilk, *lactoferrin*, actually kills *S. mutens* (Lonnerdal, 2013), and others protect and can even help re-mineralize as breastmilk deposits calcium and phosphorous on teeth. However, if your child has an enamel defect (which can happen in utero), she may be particularly vulnerable, and while breastmilk may actually be helping, she may still have decay. If your child is eating foods without brushing them off, and then lying in bed and nursing, her teeth will be subjected to the sugar in the food (all carbohydrates contain them) reacting with the bacteria in her mouth, just like anyone else. The decay-inert nature of breastmilk disappears in the presence of other foods, and it becomes decay-promoting, though without other foods present, in vitro, it resisted decay, literally for months (Erikson & Mazhari, 1999).

What about dental hygiene during the night? You work so hard to brush your child's teeth, and then she nurses several times at night. Should you be waking her up and brushing or wiping her teeth after each feeding, as some dentists recommend? Normally, there is no need. Again, studies show that breastmilk alone will not cause cavities and can, indeed, help protect from them. The important thing is to brush before the night begins so that there will be no interaction between food and bacteria during the night beyond breastmilk and, perhaps, water. Also, as breastmilk helps raise PH levels to create a less acidic mouth, it can be helpful in creating a mouth that is less hospitable to bacteria during the night (Erikson & Mazhari, 1999).

It may be near impossible during the day to keep food and breastmilk completely away from each other, but there are other factors that may set your mind at ease on this subject. First of all, bacteria require a low oral pH to thrive, and pH is typically higher during the day. Also, as a child eats, talks, and nurses during the day, his mouth will be stimulated to make saliva, which helps prevent decay (a dry mouth, especially at night, can promote decay). Lastly, an older child can sip a little water here and there to help rinse food away. If you are concerned about this daytime interaction, and your child is willing, you can brush or wipe gums after all snacks and meals. Remember, though, that despite everything you try, some decay may continue in vulnerable teeth.

So, with this information, we can see that: 1) that breastmilk and night nursing alone do *not* cause cavities, 2) that weaning (for dental reasons; you may have other reasons for considering weaning) may actually hasten decay because there is less *lactoferrin* in the mouth, and because nursing during the night can raise PH levels and re-mineralize teeth, and 3) that there may be nothing you can do for your child's teeth except to keep the mouth clean and make sure your child has a healthy diet containing foods with the necessary vitamins and minerals to help growing bodies, with as few sticky, sugary things as possible, including juices. As discussed above, you may want to examine the use of xylitol.

You may wonder if your child will automatically have dental caries in his permanent teeth because of the problems with his primary teeth. It does seem that, on a population-wide level, the probability of future problems is indeed a bit higher when children have an early history of caries (Peretz et al., 2003), but there may be reasons for this that we can control in our own lives. If the caries in the young children studied were due to damaging habits (and if they weren't breastfed–studies often do *not* examine this), or they had nutritional deficiencies, those habits and deficiencies probably continued as they grew their adult teeth and contributed to this correlation. Breastfeeding moms often observe that their children do not have continued problems, and that the health of their permanent teeth is all about lifestyle, such as hygiene and diet, just like for anyone else.

One last thought for you is that many parents, including myself, have observed that some children in their families have difficulty with decay and some do not, even when conditions (such as breastfeeding at night for several years) were similar for all of them, which further points to the idea that it is not the breastfeeding itself that is the cause. Also, moms are reporting that more recently trained dentists may be taking a different tack with caries in baby teeth, rather than just recommending weaning or extraction right off the bat. When my youngest child started to have brown spots on her teeth at the age of 3, despite a very good diet and good hygiene, our dentist (who is known for being progressive and up-to-date) said something like, "This isn't your fault. This probably happened when you were pregnant. Just keep her teeth clean and we'll leave them alone unless they begin to hurt her." Not what I was expecting, at all!

Q: I have been told that my child is too small and that I should wean. Is that true?

A: The first thing to remember about a breastfed child's weight is that if your child is growing steadily, seems healthy and happy, is peeing often enough, and is meeting developmental milestones, there is no reason to believe that they are not getting what they need from breastmilk.

Some doctors believe that eating more solid foods will make a child grow, and want parents to try to pack more in, even when a baby is not yet at the recommend age. Even if you could force your child to do this, it won't cause him to grow unless he is developmentally ready to. That's how it works. Attempting to force children to eat solids, especially at the expense of a food that is nature-made for growing bodies, usually doesn't work, and may make them resistant to solids. Early exploration of foods should be stress-free and fun; not something parents are counting on for certain results. That's a lot of pressure on everyone.

If your doctor is worried about your child's weight, you might ask him or her to look at the weight charts for the World Health Organization instead of the weight charts that doctors typically use in the U.S., which are often based on formula-fed children. Remember that there is not necessarily anything wrong with being on the lower end of the charts, in general. Health care providers sometimes want every baby to be average, but, by definition, most babies will not be. Remember also that babies' rate of growth usually slows some in the second half of their first year.

There are times, however, when worry about weight may be legitimate. When a baby has been around a certain percentage since birth and then shows a continuing trend of gaining at a much slower rate, sometimes called "falling off the curve," or has even been losing weight, there may be something wrong, especially if this is coupled with developmental delays, signs of dehydration or lethargy. If this is happening, your Lactation Consultant or your doctor will need to evaluate the situation, and may suggest breastfeeding more often, and pumping to boost supply. You may need to supplement. How you choose to do this (your pumped milk, donor milk, formula, solids if old enough) is up to you, but it may be one of those times when supplementation is simply a lesser evil. The good news is that supplementation does not mean that complete weaning is needed. Remember that you are a still a successful breastfeeding mother, even if you are not able to exclusively breastfeed at the moment. Everyone's breastfeeding journey looks different, and making sure that your baby is fed and healthy is the most important thing (Mohrbacher, 2010).

Q: I have been told that my child is too heavy and that I should wean. Is that true?

A: Again, an exclusively breastfed baby who does not have any other issues will be the size that they are naturally meant to be, and doctors should not rely too heavily on where they fall on charts, especially if they are not using the WHO charts. Some children are just naturally larger and, if they are healthy and happy, it isn't a problem.

Continuing to nurse your child will in no way cause him to be overweight, either presently or in the future. Breastfed children will not usually overfeed; they stop when they're full. In fact, studies show that breastfeeding, and especially exclusive breastfeeding for the first six months or so, helps protect children from obesity as they grow into adulthood (Centers for Disease Control and Prevention, 2007).

CHAPTER 5

Behavior and Sleep Questions

Q: : My 6-month-old daughter is so distractible, that nursing her is really difficult sometimes. I'm frustrated and wondering if weaning is a possibility for us. I know she is young, but what can I do?

A: You are not alone! "Distractible" is a word that moms often use to describe their babies at about the middle of their first year. The good news is that most moms report that this stage doesn't last long, and that your daughter is right on track developmentally. Her brain is growing, and she is going through very significant changes. The world is a new, exciting place for her, and she is compelled check it all out. That being said, it can be really frustrating for mothers to try to nurse squirmy, distracted babies. You are not alone in feeling so frustrated with it that you question your desire to continue the nursing relationship. Some mothers of super distractible babies even question whether *their babies* want to continue. Keep in mind that babies rarely self-wean before the age of one.

Most children will eat more seriously when they get hungry, and will usually have at least a few really good nursing sessions in each 24-hour period. Sometimes, babies nurse a bit more at night, during this whirlwind time, to make up for calories they miss during the day. Again, totally normal and often necessary, and this too will pass. Additionally, babies of this age are often able to get a lot of milk in a very short time, so your daughter may be getting more than you know out of those quick, acrobatic sips.

Even when mothers understand and accept this developmental stage, they often need some help to get through it. Here are some tips that have helped moms nurse distractible babies:

❋ Work in something that adds some routine to nursing, as a signal to your child that you are changing direction.

Some moms use a song or a rhyme. Some use a soft toy or blanket to help their child make the transition. Remember that anything new takes some repetition to work.

❋ Create a more controlled environment.

Not only can a special place serve as another signal in your child's routine, but it may be easier to control distractions there. You may have a bedroom in which you can draw dark curtains, put on some white noise or soft music, hold your child in a rocker or comfortable chair, and close the door to get away from the world for a bit. Some moms report that this is the only thing that has worked for them, and that they had to do this every time they really needed to nurse. It's less convenient, for sure, but, again, it doesn't last forever!

❋ "Tank up."

Nurse before you leave the house, or are going into any situation in which your child will be even more distracted (a friend coming over, a trip to the store, etc.).

❋ Wear a nursing necklace, or hold something interesting for your child to fiddle with while you are nursing.

Nursing necklaces are easily found nowadays in stores and online, and are usually non-toxic, unlike other jewelry.

✳ Don't give up too quickly on a feeding.

Sometimes mothers will put the baby down as soon as she turns away the first time. Yet, babies often want to look away (maybe with your nipple still in her mouth, so be ready with your finger to break suction), and then nurse again, over and over. If you are patient, you may be able to get a full, if interrupted, feeding in. It isn't time, yet, to replace nutritious feedings with solid food meals, so it can really pay to be persistent, but relaxed. Try to remain calm. If your baby senses that you are upset with her, it may be even more difficult to get her to focus.

✳ "Dream Feed."

I'm not sure who coined the term, but the idea is that a baby who is very sleepy, just beginning to wake, or is even completely asleep will sometimes be happy to nurse seriously when they often would not if they were awake. Some moms even find that just lying down for a feeding makes a big difference.

✳ Remind yourself, regularly, that you are doing a wonderful thing for your baby, even when it seems like she isn't appreciating it!

She still loves nursing and, soon, as she becomes able to handle nursing while checking the world out, she'll show you that she does. Repeat: "This is normal. This will pass," and breathe!

Q: My 10-month-old hasn't nursed much at all in the last two days. She pushes me away and fusses. My friend says that is how her son was when he weaned himself at 9 months. Is my baby trying to wean?

A: It sounds like you and your baby are going through a Nursing Strike. It is rare for a child of this age to intend to stop nursing, though this is what often happens as mothers misunderstand the situation.

A nursing strike is when a breastfeeding child, for whatever reason, refuses to nurse for a period of time—a few hours to a few days, usually. There can be many possible causes of a nursing strike. Sometimes, a child has had some stress or a scare when at the breast (sometimes the surprised shout of a nipple-bitten mama can do it). Sometimes, there is some pain that is not evident yet: an earache, teething pain, thrush, digestive discomfort, headache, or impending sickness that is impacting the baby's ability to nurse. There may be nasal congestion that prevents the baby from breathing well through the nose while nursing. There may even be a taste in the mother's milk that the baby doesn't like and doesn't want more of.

No matter what the situation, your baby is most likely as confused and upset about a nursing strike as you are! Something that she has always associated with comfort, enjoyment, and food (and you) is suddenly not pleasant.

So, what can you do? The first thing is to relax. Let go of any worries you may have about whether she is trying to wean and even about whether you can figure out what is going on—sometimes mothers never do find out why a strike occurred. The important thing is to provide a stable, peaceful base-of-operations; to be your normal comforting self, in other words. Even if she doesn't *seem* comforted, you are helping her and not adding to the problem.

When you are able to relax with your child, consider wearing or holding her as much as you can. Sometimes, when a child doesn't seem to be comforted by the usual methods, parents will set them down, thinking that they do not want to be held. Of course, this *is* the case every now and then, and if you set her down and she seems much happier, then use your instincts. But usually, putting down the baby does not stop the crying. The reason we continue to hold a child who is upset, even when we cannot comfort them or fix them, is to let them know that they haven't been abandoned—and won't be abandoned—even when the situation is difficult. This message is important and their security in knowing that you will be there for them, no matter what, will stand you in good stead as they grow! Additionally, being in constant contact with your child may stimulate her to nurse, and will ensure that you don't miss cues as they arise.

Another helpful technique is to offer the breast often and at times you might not normally. Many mothers report that a child who will not nurse when awake will nurse well when just waking, half-asleep, or even completely asleep. You can also see if a change of venue or style will help. Some moms find that a striking nurser will nurse outside, or in the car, or when walking or dancing around. Like the distracted nurser, a quiet dark room may help with a strike. Lastly, it can be helpful to talk to other nursing moms about how they handled a nursing strike. If you are overwhelmed and need to talk, consider calling La Leche League or Breastfeeding USA, or any other group of supportive breastfeeding moms you may be a part of.

Q. My mother says she weaned me abruptly when I bit her at 6 months old. So, of course, I am really worried about biting! What do I do? I don't really want to wean, but I can't imagine nursing a child who bites me.

A: Most babies bite at some point. Usually, the first bite is just due to playing/ experimenting or to teething pain, though there can be other reasons. Babies don't intend to hurt their mothers and biting is rarely more than a temporary problem. A biting baby is not intending to wean and biting is not considered a reason that mothers need to wean, especially as this too will pass.

If your baby does bite, it can be helpful to have some ideas of how to handle this before it happens, so you don't feel totally ambushed. Some techniques that other mothers have used and most experts recommend are:

✱ Keep your cool!

It can be difficult, but it is really important. Some moms have reported a nursing strike occurring after their screaming scared the baby, so there is good reason to stay calm. Additionally, stress at the breast can cause fussiness and anxiety. However, sometimes we just have no control over our outbursts when bitten, so we all just do the best we can. If you do scare your baby, be sure to quickly comfort and reconnect. You can work on doing better the next time, if it happens again.

❋ Take the baby off the breast, breaking suction if needed, and hold her on your lap (some moms of babies able to sit unsupported will set them down) for a few seconds.

Often, this is enough for the baby to get the message that nursing and biting don't mix, though you may have to do it several times. You might calmly say "no bite" or something similar. Your baby may be upset, and this isn't a punishment, just a message, so it is important that this break doesn't last more than a few seconds. Your baby will probably be grateful to nurse again, and that may be all that is needed.

❋ Pay attention and be ready to act.

If it seems like your baby is going through a biting "stage," and more intervention is needed, watch your baby while nursing. The mechanics of breastfeeding are such that it is almost impossible for a baby to bite while she is feeding because her tongue has to stick out over her bottom teeth to provide an effective suck. Biting usually happens when the active nursing is done and experimenting begins.

Sometimes, mothers will end the feeding when the active nursing ends by breaking suction with her finger and moving on to some other activity, or she may allow some extra sucking in case the baby is trying to get another letdown or taking a break. Be vigilant and ready to break suction if a bite happens, or seems like it might. Your close attention may also help you figure out what is causing the biting or what the pattern is.

❋ Find an alternative for baby to bite on.

If you suspect your baby's biting is due to teething, you might consider having something nearby that they *can* bite on. Some moms use a washcloth (sometimes frozen, so it is cold) or other teether, and then, if bitten, will calmly stop breastfeeding and give the baby the alternative, putting the baby back on as soon as she shows she wants to nurse. This gives the message about what is okay to bite, and what is not.

These are just a few things you can do to help with biting, and you can find out many more by talking with other breastfeeding mothers. Remember that this will probably be a very short-lived problem, if you experience it at all, and that most breastfeeding mothers have been through it. You don't have to allow fear of biting to end your lovely nursing relationship.

Q: My child does not seem interested in solid foods. Would weaning help?

A: Much of how babies interact with solid food just depends on who they are. Some children love solids from the get-go, and some wait a long time before they do much more than taste them. We don't always know why this is, but we do know that tension around solid foods tends to cause trouble, and a relaxed manner towards them doesn't.

Unfortunately, this is an area where others may pressure you, wanting your child eating three square meals a day plus snacks as soon as possible. But nursing moms know that their children get great nutrition from breastmilk, even as they move into toddlerhood, though they may need to make sure vitamin D and iron levels are good. Most of these moms don't worry too much about the exact amount of solid food that their babies are eating; they just offer nutritious foods regularly and calmly.

How your child would eat if you were to wean for this purpose is unknown. What is known is that there are no solid foods as nutrient-dense as your milk, and that none of them do the myriad of things your milk can. Furthermore, if your child is under a year of age, she will still need a breastmilk substitute, not just solids. Many moms find it easier to keep nursing while negotiating solids, rather than switch to formula.

Experts believe that we can trust our children to know what foods, and how much of them they need, if they are offered healthy, age-appropriate choices, including breastmilk. The book, *My Child Won't Eat! How to Enjoy Mealtimes Without Worry* by Carlos Gonzalez, is helpful to many parents in your situation, and while you may not change your kid's eating habits much, you'll feel a lot better about them, and feel more confident in talking to others about this issue.

Q: I have been told that my baby will sleep more if I wean her. Is that true?

A: It is easy for others around us to turn every challenge we have as a parent into a problem that needs to be solved. Most breastfeeding and gentle-parenting experts agree that the stages that babies and children go through are not problems; they are developmentally appropriate and instinctive behaviors, whether we understand them or not. In La Leche League, it is often said that babies cannot manipulate you. They do not have the capacity to ask for something that they don't truly need, and this includes sleeping/waking and night nursing.

Some babies don't need many night feedings, and some wake several times to nurse for quite some time. Neither of these is wrong and much of this variation is be due to their mothers' natural "milk storage capacity" (babies who can get a lot at one time may nurse less often and vice-versa), among other things. You can feel confident that you are doing the right thing by meeting your baby's nursing needs during the night. She will not learn bad habits. She will be able to "soothe herself" in the future. Generations of mothers who parented as needed during the night, and whose children are now healthy adult sleepers offer great proof of this (Mohrbacher, 2014b).

There is a lot of pressure on parents these days to get their babies sleeping through the night as soon as possible, and lots of misinformation claiming that babies should not need their parents at night after a few months of age. However, if your baby isn't ready to do this, you are not teaching her anything except to give up on her needs. Translation: You won't be there for her, so she should shut down. What happens in babies' brains and bodies as they do this can be stressful, to say the least, and there is evidence that there may be more long-term harm done than short-term good (as defined by a bit more parental sleep). There is science behind this, and sharing this with others in your life may help them realize that you accept your baby where she is, and want to meet her needs. When she is older and ready, unless there is some underlying problem, she will sleep more. For now, know that a baby who wakes to nurse is showing one sign of being very healthy and attached (Ockwell-Smith, 2014).

But would your baby would sleep more if you weaned? A young baby who is night-weaned or completely weaned may or may not sleep more and, if they do, may be "shutting down," as discussed. Additionally, weaned babies often still need to eat or be comforted during the night (and, indeed, waking for a child under 6 months old can be a safety mechanism), so you would have to consider what you would feed your baby, and what other tools you would use to respond to her needs, if you weaned.

An older child who wakes a lot ("a lot" being relative to each family) and asks to nurse may or may not sleep more when weaned or night-weaned. It really depends a great deal on the individual child and the reason behind the waking: hunger, food sensitivities, discomfort, etc. Remember, even if you choose to night-wean, and must meet needs differently, your child still has legitimate needs. Mothers who choose to wean for this reason should have some backup ideas in place to soothe their children, and should consider finding the source of waking if it continues. Mothers who try night weaning often find that it works best when the child is old enough to understand what the mother is asking of them (Mohrbacher, 2012). If you would like more information on night-weaning, please see the section on "partial weaning" in Chapter 10.

All that aside, moms do need sleep. As brief as this time is, it can feel like torture when you are tired. There are many helpful ideas that do not require that parents ignore or try to change their babies' needs. The book, *Sweet Sleep: Nighttime and Naptime Strategies for the Breastfeeding Family* by Diane Wiessinger, Diana West, Linda J. Smith, and Teresa Pitman is a new favorite among breastfeeding families, and *The Baby Sleep Book: The Complete Guide to a Good Night's Rest for the Whole Family* by William Sears, Martha Sears, Robert Sears, and James Sears, and *The No-Cry Sleep Solution: Gentle Ways to Help Your Baby Sleep Through the Night* by Elizabeth Pantley, are old favorites.

Some Strategies That Parents Use to Get More Sleep

✸ Tank up.

It can help to make sure that children are getting full nursing sessions in during the night, rather than quick suckles and back to sleep. Moms will nudge and reawaken a little until their children have nursed for a good amount of time, perhaps massaging and doing breast compressions to keep the milk flowing and to make sure their babies get all the fat in the milk that they need to be satiated.

✸ Choose when the child has longest period of sleep.

Often, the longest period of a child's sleep, 4 or 5 hours, is when parents haven't even gone to bed yet. Soon after the mom falls asleep, the baby wakes, and the shorter cycles begin. Some moms have been able to switch this longer period to coincide with their own first hours of sleep by waking the baby just before they go to bed and encouraging a full nursing session then. It may take a few repetitions, but it can be worth it.

✸ Change the environment.

For some families, this can mean adopting safe bedsharing. For others, it can mean moving from bedsharing to a different co-sleeping arrangement. Barbara Higham, on the "Women's Health Today" blog post entitled "Sleep Like a Baby" defines bedsharing and co-sleeping like this: "The term "bedsharing" implies a baby sharing an adult bed with one or both parents. The term "co-sleeping" implies a baby is sleeping in close proximity to an adult caregiver, not necessarily in the same bed" (Higham, 2017). This "close proximity" is still very important for your child and your breastfeeding relationship, so any changes will work best if it is maintained.

Parents who feel strongly either way about bedsharing can have difficulty with the idea of switching. But sometimes they find that a change helps everyone get more sleep.

✻ Work on "latching off" and being able to move away after nursing.

When children won't let the breast go after nursing, it can be difficult to get enough sleep. For help with this, please see the following question in this chapter that addresses "latching off."

Q: My child won't latch off at night without waking up, and I can't leave the bed without her waking! How can I get her to let me go?

A: These are difficulties that many parents face, whether bedsharing, or in some other co-sleeping arrangement.

Here are some things that some mothers have found helpful for "latching off" and moving away from their babies.

✻ Pick your moment.

Early on, while nursing my children, I noticed certain sleep requirements that had to be met before I could latch them off easily. I began to call this their "magic ratio." As I worked with mothers and shared these observations over the years, many of them reported that they were able to use them successfully as well.

Most mothers know that humans have sleep cycles, but they rarely think of this in relation to their babies. They usually assume that their babies are in a deep enough sleep when they stop nursing actively, and they latch them off, only to find that they wake and want to actively nurse again.

The key is to observe your child. For a few nights, just watch. What does his breathing and sucking cycle look like? When *is* he okay with being detached from the nipple? When is he not? From my experience, and what many mothers have told me after observation, I believe that most children have a certain place in the cycle that means they are truly asleep and can be latched off. What if this is ignored and the mom tries too early? The cycle is interrupted and must begin again.

The cycle of breathing/sucking after active nursing is finished may look like this: at first, maybe four or five deep breaths to four or five seconds of fluttery, weak sucking. Then it may stretch to seven or eight breaths, and two or three seconds of sucking. Sooner or later, they reach their personal "magic ratio," which usually varies only when they are sick or in a growth spurt. For one, it might be 12 breaths to one second of light sucking. For another, 10 breaths to two seconds. When they got to this place, moms can use a finger to gently break suction, and they will stay asleep. You might try this observation of your child's cycle to see when you can safely latch off. It may be that, like many of us, you are anxious to do other things and are just latching off too early.

❋ Get them used to the feeling.

Another technique that some mothers say worked for them too (which is somewhat opposite of the previous one) is intentionally breaking suction with their finger as soon as necessary, active nursing is finished, leaving the nipple near, and allowing their child to immediately latch back on. Then, a few seconds later, they do it again (and then again) and, often, the child will give up after a few of these repetitions, too sleepy to keep trying. Some moms report that the child turns away from them. Akin to this, some moms will simply press a bit with a finger near the side of the mouth to re-stimulate sucking until the baby gets tired of it and latches off. Certainly, you wouldn't want to do either of these if your baby was upset or annoyed by them, and always, you will want to wait until they are truly finished eating.

✸ Use movement.

When a baby wakes easily because of the movements and sounds of others, many mothers respond by remaining as still and quiet as possible at all times, which can feel very oppressive. But some moms find that it can be more helpful to get their children used to sleeping through movement, and a little noise and change. They may begin shifting around and making soft noises while nursing to get their baby used to these things, wherever they will eventually be sleeping.

If bedsharing, moms might ask a sibling or their partner to get on or off the bed once the baby seems asleep while still latched on, hoping to get their child used to movement without associating it with nursing being taken away. If putting in a crib or co-sleeper, moms might stand up, and then sit down while still nursing. They might move to a different place or position. Still, others will do little things: moving the child's arm or leg, holding a hand and then letting it go, stroking hair, tickling a foot, talking softly, all while nursing. After several days or weeks, some moms find that when they latch off, making sure their children are deeply asleep, their movements are much less disturbing to their children.

✸ Substitute a finger for the breast.

Some mothers find that their children are willing to accept their pinky finger (pad up, clean and with trimmed nails) as a substitute for their breasts after active nursing has ended. They are happy to let go of the breast as long as they can keep sucking for a bit. This doesn't immediately solve the problem of you wanting to move away and do other things, but it can provide you with a way to change your physical environment and position a bit, and some children will let go of the finger sucking more easily than the breast when their sucking need is met. You may think this two-step process of latching off works better for you than just trying to remove yourself all at once.

These techniques come from observation and conversational reporting, not from any studies or recommendations from experts. However, there isn't a lot out there from experts on ways to latch off or move away from children with compassion, so these may be helpful to you.

CHAPTER 6

Toddlers and Older Children

Q: My 14-month-old is only nursing once or twice per day for a few minutes. Does this mean that he might be trying to wean?

A: It is normal for an older toddler or young child to begin to nurse less as they become more interested in the world around them. This is a natural part of the weaning process, but it does not mean that your child is trying to wean immediately and completely. It means that the process has begun, and is progressing naturally, per your child's needs. If you don't have any overwhelming reason for the process to be sped up, then there is nothing you need to change.

Please note that this situation is very different than a "nursing strike," which is when a child has been nursing normally suddenly refuses to nurse, sometimes for several days. There are many reasons why this happens, including painful teething, upset stomach, or emotional trauma, but often mothers believe that their child no longer wants to nurse, and they end up weaning them before they are ready.

Q: My 1-year-old is difficult to nurse in public, often making me show more than I would like. What can I do? Does this mean she is too old to nurse?

A: It isn't abnormal for a toddler or older child to be a little harder to nurse in public, especially if they are pulling your shirt up, or changing sides constantly. This isn't a sign of being ready to wean, in and of itself. It is a sign of their great enthusiasm for life, their ease with nursing (they are so proficient that they can do gymnastics while nursing), and the exciting developmental leaps they are making. That doesn't change the fact that it can be disconcerting to nurse this way, and you may need some ideas for how to handle this new nursing behavior.

From your child's perspective, your body and hers seem almost like one, and she may not understand yet, that you and she are actually separate human beings! Surprise: the mom is a person, and she has preferences about her body! Teaching your child how to behave toward your body helps her learn compassion for others, and to speak up for her own needs as she sees your example. That doesn't mean that you need to be harsh with her, or expect immediate or unreasonable results. There is no quick fix for a developmental stage. It does mean that you can begin a dialogue with her that will pay off over time.

Some Ideas That May Help in the Short- and Long-Term

❋ Be clear about your expectations.

Children can understand what we say long before they can have a real discussion, so don't feel afraid to talk. It can be helpful to let your child know your expectations in simple language, and give him some acceptable options rather than just saying "no." For example, if your child often lifts your shirt in public, you might tell her something like, "Mommy's breasts are only for private. I don't want my shirt pulled up so other people can see them. You can nurse while I hold my shirt down, or you can have a snack or a drink instead." At first, he may resist this, but the idea will sink in over time.

✸ Be preventative.

One of the most helpful things is to review your expectations and plans *every time* you go out, *before* you reach your destination: "Remember, when we are playing at the park, when you nurse, you have to leave my shirt down. If you don't want that, you can eat some cheese or have some water (or whatever you've come up with). Okay?" You might want to make sure he hears you by getting an "okay" in response, or at least some eye contact. Like everything else, this transition will take a little getting used to. You may find that he agrees in the car and then forgets when you are at the park, and that's okay. It takes time, but it does work.

✸ See what *you* can change to help the situation.

Some moms find a renewed interest in specialized nursing clothing as their children move into athletic nursing. Moms also find it helpful to notice when and where your child's nursing behavior is a problem. Is the activity boring to your child? Do you stay a little too long? Do other things take your attention? Is your child overwhelmed? These things can all make your child want to nurse more, and changing how you do things may assist them in having better nursing manners.

✸ Distract.

Many kids will ask to nurse, but will happily do just about anything else that is fun, especially if mom or dad is jumping up to do it with them. This can be a great way to avoid saying "no" to nursing, and the meltdown that can come along with it.

✸ Practice at home.

Diane Bengson mentions some ways that mothers of older nurslings handle issues of privacy and criticism in her book, *How Weaning Happens*. Regarding children who ask to nurse in ways that can be uncomfortable, she says,

> If you value nursing discreetly in public, you will want to be
> consistent about nursing discreetly at home as well. This may

mean that you require your child to "Ask with words" rather than grab your breasts, or stick his head under your shirt, even at home. It may mean that you begin to use a "code word" for nursing so that only you and your child know what is going on (Bengson, 1999, p. 105).

Remember, other people are more oblivious than we realize, but if they seem disapproving or hostile, they can move or look away from you. Yes, it is often a new experience in United States culture for folks to see even a newborn nursing in public. That doesn't mean that you are doing something wrong. In fact, the more people witness mothers nursing their children, the less it will seem strange, so you are helping future mothers and babies every time you nurse in public.

Some women never feel okay nursing in public because of religious beliefs or personal discomfort. They may always feel more comfortable finding private places to nurse, and this is a personal choice. They should not be made to feel that they *must* nurse in public.

Q: I have been told that a child "this age" is only nursing for comfort. Is that true?

A: Whatever the age of your nursling, there are benefits and, yes, comfort is one of them. Even if it was the *only* one, there would still be great value in nursing even though, in our society, the need for comfort (and the giving of it) is often seen as coddling, dangerous, and self-indulgent. A child's need for comfort is significant, and a mother's ability to comfort him is part of her magic. It's a great gift, not a bad habit.

We can't protect our children from everything in life, but what if just the knowledge that other people can be a source of comfort is a help to them as they grow? What if it makes a huge difference in their future life? Your child is learning that connections are comfort. She is also learning that she can provide comfort for others.

Comfort *isn't* the only thing that nursing gives your toddler or older child. Sometimes health care providers, or others, tell you that your milk does nothing, nutritionally or otherwise, once your child turns 1. It's as though this magical food is good one moment, and not the next. After all, it's "just comfort." In reality, the nutritional and other benefits of your milk actually change as your child grows. The milk you give to a 1-year-old is not the milk you gave to your infant. It is now designed for the needs of an active toddler or preschooler. This doesn't mean that your child won't need solid foods as she grows. It just means that your milk, and the time at your breast, isn't suddenly useless. For a list of continued benefits of nursing beyond a year, please see the following question.

Q: What are the benefits of breastfeeding longer than a year?

A: Most of us know the benefits of breastfeeding in general, but there are continued and additional benefits of nursing beyond the minimum recommendations.

Here is a list of just some of the many benefits:

❋ Connection and comfort

Rather than needing us less, toddlers need us differently. They love exploring the world, but need to connect quickly with mom when they are hurt, overwhelmed, scared, or tired. Nursing and a cuddle forces us to stop and give a focused moment of attention when they need it. Certainly, there are lots of amazing non-nursing moms who do this too, but for some of us (often distracted and busy), nursing is a vital connection.

❋ Convenience

Mothers of nursing toddlers will tell you that it's fabulous to be able to change a situation (in a store, at a gathering, etc.) from bad to good with just a quick nursing session. Many call nursing a "reset button."

✴ Nutrition

The milk you give your toddler or preschooler is different than when she was a baby. It is amazingly and specifically designed for the needs of an older child. Rather than doing nothing, as some people say, your milk still provides nutritional benefits (vitamins, minerals, fats, etc.), and many of those benefits are long-lasting, as they help grow strong bodies.

✴ Immunity

Again, the immunological properties of your milk change according to the needs of your older child. The protection that you give just by nursing is still very valuable.

✴ Independence

I'm quoting Dr. Jack Newman and Edith Kernerman (2009) again because I love what they say about this: "The child who breastfeeds until he weans himself (usually from 2 to 4 years), is usually *more* independent, and, perhaps, more importantly, *more secure* in his independence…"

I think many moms of older nurslings would agree with this, whether or not they eventually have a child-led weaning or not.

✴ Sickness

When a child has a stomach bug and can't keep anything down, many breastfeeding mothers are relieved that their children will still nurse, lowering their chances of dehydration.

✴ Future health for both child and mother

The evidence shows that many of the health benefits of breastfeeding are compounded the longer you nurse. We know many of the benefits for children, but there are lots for moms too. For example, the Mayo clinic says in regard to mothers, "Extended breastfeeding—as well as breastfeeding for 12 months or more cumulatively in life—has been shown to reduce the risk of breast cancer, ovarian cancer, rheumatoid arthritis, high blood pressure, heart disease, and diabetes" (Mayo Clinic Staff, 2015).

Q: I am not enjoying nursing a toddler anymore. When CAN I quit?

A: Humans have been nursing through the toddler and preschool years for a long, long time. However, some moms of older nurslings start to feel like they don't have the time or energy to take care of themselves the way that they want to. They feel resentment as their child becomes a toddler, and they see nursing as part of this constant demand on them and their bodies.

Parenting a toddler is difficult, and can be overwhelming for anyone, whether breastfeeding or not. Many mothers have never learned how to take of themselves, or how to make self-care a priority in their families. Moms who make a special effort to help everyone in their family understand how much they need time to themselves to rest, create, or socialize (or whatever rejuvenates them) usually find that they resent *all* of their mom duties less, and that they feel more like a whole person than "just a mom."

Sometimes moms need some personal counseling to learn to speak up or figure out how to take care of themselves. Sometimes they find great benefit in switching perspectives, if they can. So much of how we feel is in the constant dialogue we have with ourselves, and the way we look at things. For example, "I'm so tired, I can't take it anymore" when, in contrast, some moms see breastfeeding sessions as their breaks. They feel that the other parts of parenting require them to be up, doing, planning, entertaining, and other tiring things. Breastfeeding? They get to sit. They get to reconnect with a child who never slows down except to nurse. They get to read a book, maybe, or talk on the phone for a few minutes. Perhaps they finally get to sit and breathe or pray or meditate. Sometimes a shift in perspective can be all it takes to go from feeling resentful to feeling grateful.

As far as the "When CAN I quit" question goes, it sounds like to are worried that you will be required to nurse for longer than you think you want to. If that is true, let me remind you of the lovely wording of the AAP recommendations regarding nursing duration; "1 year or longer as *mutually desired by mother and infant*" (italics added) (Eidelman & Schandler, 2012). If you have strong feelings that you don't want to nurse anymore, you may owe it to your future self, and to your child, to try to figure out what those feelings are about, and whether weaning will solve them. It may be that you are *not* mutually desiring to continue breastfeeding, and you may be ready to begin the process of weaning. This does not mean you are a bad mother. Negative feelings about parts of motherhood are not rare, nor are they wrong; they are just feelings and they are telling you something. Remember that you have already given your child the amazing gift of breastfeeding, and you will continue to be a loving and devoted mother, as you always have been, when you wean. For ideas of how to begin weaning, please see Section Three of this book.

Q: I feel terribly emotional when I think about weaning. I had planned to stop at a year, but now I can't imagine taking it away from my baby. What can I do?

A: You aren't alone in feeling this way. The nursing relationship is an expression of deep love, and sometimes the ability to breastfeed is hard-won, a victory of the highest order, and moms can worry that weaning is a curtain coming down on what has been a beautiful time.

Remember that this lovely time doesn't really end. Whenever the actual physical act of breastfeeding ceases, the closeness you have created, the bond of trust, the instincts you have honed are here for you both forever. In many cases, weaning is a gradual progression: less of an ending and more of an expression of growth that doesn't conclude until you and your child are ready. Assuming your child has already been sampling solid food, the weaning journey has already begun, probably somewhat painlessly.

You are not hurting anything by continuing to nurse, or even by nursing until your child is ready to wean on his own, as many mothers do around the world. This is often called a "child-led" or "natural" weaning: a grow-out-of-it process, rather than one in which there is a schedule or expected age of weaning.

Here is a lovely quote from the Mayo Clinic website:

> Worldwide, babies are weaned on average between ages 2 and 4. In some cultures, breastfeeding continues until children are age 6 or 7. In other parts of the world, however, extended breastfeeding is less common, and can sometimes provoke uninformed, negative reactions.
>
> How long you breastfeed is up to you and your baby. If loved ones—and even strangers—share their opinions about when to wean, remind them that the decision is yours. Try not to worry about what other people think. Instead, trust your instincts.
>
> Extended breastfeeding can be an intimate way to continue nurturing your baby. If you're considering extended breastfeeding, think about what's best for both you and your baby—and enjoy this special time together (Mayo Clinic Staff, 2015).

CHAPTER 7

Working and Pumping

Note: If you are experiencing extraordinary difficult or hostile working circumstances, please see discussion of this topic in Chapter 2.

Q: **I will be traveling quite a bit with my new job. I would like to keep nursing, but I feel like I may have to wean. What can I do?**

A: Unless you have a specific desire to wean, there is no need to wean just because you will be away from your child. Of course, being away for several days when you have a young baby might be difficult, though mothers have certainly done it by making sure that their baby has enough pumped milk for the feedings they will miss, and by pumping as often as they can when away. When you have a toddler or older child who is still nursing, it can be a little easier, though they will probably still need some pumped milk, and you will certainly want to pump while away to keep your supply up, and because mastitis would not be a fun travel companion! Many babies and children are happy to pick up with nursing when their mothers return from an extended absence, though some will not.

Here are some things to consider:

✸ Feelings

You may be a bit of a mess without your baby, especially at first. So many moms get excited, imagining how luxurious it will feel to relax by themselves in a hotel room, but end up feeling lost and sad. Your baby may be a bit of a mess without you, *or* she may be totally fine, which can be even harder to take. Don't worry; she still loves and needs you. She's just got good caregivers and a certain kind of personality.

You may feel like you have a hard time concentrating on work when you are away and worried about your baby. Being away in this age of easy-to-use technology is so different than when even the telephone was expensive to use long distance. Some moms are able to video chat with their babies or get regular video updates of them, which can help.

You may feel guilty. You may worry that you aren't a good mom, or that others will think you aren't. Just know this: your concern about this situation is proof that you *are* a good mom, and are devoted to your baby. No one else understands your situation and the choices you must make, and if anyone is unkind, then their opinions probably don't matter much.

Reconnection with your child might not be immediate. Depending on age, babies don't always understand the changes as you come and go and, even when everyone does their best, it can be hard on them. Sometimes, when you return, they ignore you, or act like they don't want to see you. Don't worry. Be patient and let them acclimate. They will reconnect. They still love you, and do need you.

✸ Practical matters

Do you have enough milk stored to cover feedings plus some extra in case of spills or growth spurts? Most breastfeeding moms don't want to have to add in formula while they are away, if they can help it, as it can be hard on babies' systems.

Do your caregivers understand and support the breastfeeding

relationship? There are ways that they can help you beyond just being with your baby while you are not. As mentioned previously, they can help you video chat with your baby, or talk on the phone with you so that she can see you and/or hear your voice. They can feed her in a way that more closely mimics breastfeeding, such as "paced feeding," using "slow-flow nipples," and following your baby's cues (Wiessinger et al., 2010).

Do you have the information you need to succeed? The book, *Breastfeeding in Combat Boots: A Survival Guide to Successful Breastfeeding While Serving in the Military* by Robin Roche-Paull, is loved by many working mothers, even those who aren't in the military, for its excellent information about breastfeeding through longer-than-usual separation. Websites, such as LLLI.org and BreastfeedingUSA.org, are also great resources for good information about travelling and separation.

❃ Your child's feelings

You don't need anyone to tell you, I am sure, how much your child loves snuggling and nursing with her mom. She is going to have feelings about these longer separations, and she will need you and other caregivers to accept her emotions as normal, and let her process them, no matter what her age. That takes patience, compassion, and physical connection. If she is clingy while you are gone, or when you come back, that is normal. If the adults in her life give her the physical and emotional support she is asking for, they won't be teaching her bad habits, or making her dependent. They will be providing security and breeding trust, two things that will help her feel safe while she goes through separation that she can't understand and has no say about.

✳ Support

Do you have support from mothers who have been in your situation? Getting to ask questions of moms who have been exactly where you are now, and who have shared your concerns, is priceless. There are many groups, both online and in person, that can help you find other working/ breastfeeding moms. In my experience, these moms are more than happy to help each other and you. Here are some: La Leche League, Breastfeeding USA, and Mom2Mom Global (U.S. Military). There are also many Facebook groups specifically for working/breastfeeding mothers.

Note: In the past, LLL Leaders did not have much experience supporting working mothers. This has changed greatly in recent times, with most groups realizing the importance of working and breastfeeding, and welcoming mothers and Leaders who have this experience. Our local, Southwestern Virginia, USA group contains more working mothers than not, and half of our 6 Leaders are working mothers.

Q: I am going back to work in a month and my baby still nurses a lot. My friend says it will be so much easier if I wean now, especially for the daycare workers. Is this true?

A: Your friend is trying to help, of course, but you should know that many women have continued to nurse their babies while returning to work, and that their numbers are increasing every day. Working and mothering is commonplace now, and mothers continue to nurse because they cherish this relationship and the easy reconnection it provides. Also, considering that most moms in the U.S. go back to work when their child is under 6 months of age, continuing to nurse may be very important for both you and your child.

Here are some specific practices or items that are helpful to moms transitioning back into the workplace:

✸ A good pump and all the parts needed

Not all pumps are created equal, so you may want to do some research.

✸ A good plan

Speak with employers long before the return date, if possible, and explain clearly and simply what is needed (travel considerations, pumping times, milk storage). This can be integral to a trouble-free transition.

✸ Good support

Whether you have a family member who can watch your child, or you are placing your child in daycare, some education about how to care for a breastfeeding child may be in order. Your care provider may need to read about paced feeding and the unique ways that breastfed children eat, as compared to those who are formula-fed, or exclusively bottle-fed. Your care provider may need to be understanding about any difficulty your attached child has as he adjusts to being away from you.

Good support may also include joining a breastfeeding support group in which there are moms who understand the unique needs of working-breastfeeding moms and babies. Moms who have been where you are now are often very eager to pass on what they have learned, and to support you in your journey.

✸ A good understanding of how breastfeeding may change for you

It is very common for babies to "reverse cycle." This means that your baby may not feed during the day as often as he would when with you. He may, instead, nurse more when with you, including at night, making the calories up when he can breastfeed. Rest assured that this is natural. Many moms report that they enjoy the closeness and reconnection of evening, and even night nursing.

Also, this night nursing, especially with a child under a year of age, will protect your milk supply, which can be vulnerable when you are away and pumping during the day. No pump can take the place of your child when it comes to supply and demand, and your child instinctively knows this, and will attempt to stimulate you more at night and in the early morning, when the hormones that cause us to make milk are at their highest (Mohrbacher, 2010).

For additional support, the books, *Breastfeeding and Working Made Simple* by Nancy Mohrbacher and *Nursing Mother, Working Mother: The Essential Guide to Breastfeeding Your Baby Before and After You Return to Work* by Gale Pryor and Kathleen Huggins are great resources that can help you feel prepared for this new phase of your breastfeeding relationship.

Q: I have been pumping at work for almost a year now, and I am so tired of it! I love nursing, but I can't take much more pumping! Should I wean?

A: There is no doubt that working and breastfeeding can be complicated, and that many factors come into play. Some moms find pumping to be very easy with supportive employers and co-workers, and the enjoyment of a bit of quiet time every few hours. Others have a much harder time finding a time and place to pump, and may find pumping itself to be difficult, even at the best of times. The amazing thing, to me, is how many moms make it work!

If you aren't having issues with nursing but simply with pumping, there is no reason that you need to wean completely, if you don't want to. More than a few mothers find themselves at a place where they are ready to end the relationship with their pump, though not with nursing in general. Most of the time, it is perfectly okay to do this, as long as your child is old enough to have other foods while you are away from them, and you haven't had any major supply issues (and even then, you may be able to make it work if you are willing to go slowly and assess the situation regularly).

The primary factors to consider, of course, are the age and personality of your child. If your child is over a year old, and happy to eat solids when with care providers, it may be easy for him to switch to other foods and drinks. However, if your child still finds a great deal of comfort in knowing that he has your milk when away from you, or he is not that interested in solids, he may not be ready for this transition. Don't despair! Many times, kids who aren't ready for something right now are just fine with it a short time later. Relax, observe, and see what you can do to promote his favorite healthy foods in preparation for the future.

Even if your child is happy to eat and drink other foods, if you have dealt with serious or chronic supply issues, pumping may be doing a lot more than just providing milk for your child. It may also be instrumental in keeping up the demand side of the supply-and-demand nature of breastfeeding. In this situation, you will want to be very thoughtful about how you change things.

If you have dealt with chronic plugged ducts or mastitis, pumping while you are away from your child may be helping you prevent them. This doesn't mean that you can't taper off, but it may mean that you will want to keep a watch on things and go even more slowly than some mothers would. Even mothers who have never had these problems can experience them if they abruptly wean from the pump, so always remember to be patient and go slowly.

Like any kind of weaning, you will be using some version of cutting pumping sessions, whether completely or gradually. If you cut out a feeding, experts Nancy Mohrbacher and Kathleen Kendall-Tackett recommend taking several days to get used to this change before you consider cutting another. You can "pump just to comfort" (stopping as soon as you feel relief, rather than pumping fully), or hand express (also "just to comfort") if needed (2010, p. 173).

How to Cut Out a Pumping Session

This can be done by completely removing a pumping, all at once, and watching your body's reaction carefully. You can also cut a pumping session more slowly over time by deferring it. Just like it sounds, moms push their next pumping forward a bit, eventually bringing it close enough to the next one to drop it. This version of removing a pumping can be easier on your body because it is more gradual, so mothers who are prone to mastitis or plugged ducts may prefer it. Another gentle-on-the-body method can be to reduce pumping time. This is a commonly used method for dropping a breastfeeding session, and it is even easier to implement with a pump because you don't need any agreement from a child to do it. It is a gradual process, and can be applied to one session at a time, or to all of them equally. Mothers stop pumping a short time, perhaps just a minute or two, before they normally would, seeing how they feel, and giving ample time to get used to it before shortening more. Eventually, one or more sessions will be short enough to discontinue altogether.

Weaning from the pump need not change your breastfeeding relationship at home. Happily, many working mothers find that as their children grow older, their bodies easily adjust to making milk only when they are with them and can nurse.

How to Make Weaning Work for Your Family

CHAPTER 8

Making Plans

Your child (probably) has one big talent, and it's breastfeeding. Think of the one big talent you have (maybe you are lucky enough to have many) that you really value. Now, imagine that someone is telling you that that talent has to end. There's no other way, no way to avoid it; it will end. Most of us would want to have a say in how that ending comes about. We'd want acknowledgement of how important that talent was to us. We'd want comfort and love as we move away from it. We can do this for our kids. We can give them the same consideration that we would hope for and, in the process, model empathy and kindness for them.

In this chapter, I offer you four steps for creating a compassionate weaning plan. The actual weaning plans of families will differ and be very individual. Your loving weaning may take several weeks, months, or even years, depending on your family's needs and your weaning approach, and that is okay. From your child's perspective, and your body's perspective, the slower, the better.

Note: If you are considering weaning a child younger than age 1, there are special considerations you will want to be aware of, though the four steps and many of the techniques can still be applied. Considerations are discussed in the following section: creating a weaning plan for a child from 6 months to 1 year of age.

The Four Steps

1. Relax
2. Observe
3. Make a Simple, Clear, and Flexible Plan
4. Implement and Evaluate

Step One: Relax

The first thing to do is to *relax*. Unless you are in dire circumstances, nothing must happen this exact moment, and parents usually work best with a few breaths, a clear head, and some good information.

Keep breathing. Remember that all children wean, and yours will too. Don't worry about those around you unless they are kind and supportive of your choices and your bond with your child. You can do this, in partnership and in love.

Step Two: Observe

Take a bit of time to really observe your child's habits and personality, as well as your own feelings and needs, and the present dynamic in your household. Don't worry about them; your job is just to watch so that you can create a weaning plan that will work for your child and family. Understanding the needs of everyone involved will help you do that.

Don't get too frustrated if things vary during the observation phase. Just like adults, children are able to do things some days, and not others, for all kinds of reasons. Learning to accept how your child's abilities vary is a great skill for you to have now, and for the rest of parenting. This is not going backward; you are still observing. More active work can come later.

Observing Your Child

Here are a few examples of questions you might ask while observing your child and your nursing relationship.

Is your child very attached to certain nursing sessions and less so to others?

Most children over a certain age have nursing sessions that they seem to need more than others, both for hunger and for comfort and, usually, these sessions are the very last ones dropped. Often, they occur first thing in the morning, and last thing before bedtime and naptime. Cessation of these for children who aren't ready can lead to a lot of agitation and insecurity and, possibly, a lot more work for parents. You can make a note of when nursing is most important to your child and resolve to keep these protected for now. Remember, too, that comfort (among other benefits that nursing continues to provide) is a very legitimate need for a child, and is not less important than the food that you provide for her.

Is your child easily distractible, tending to choose play over breastfeeding, depending on the time of day?

As children grow, they become much more interested in the world around them and will often choose other exciting activities over nursing unless hungry, tired, or otherwise in need. It doesn't mean that they *intend* not to nurse; it is just that they are easily distracted and you may be able to use this to your advantage. Observe when this seems to happen regularly and naturally, and when you are ready, you may find that these are the easiest nursing sessions to modify. Remember that some children are naturally less distractible than others, and that this will change as they grow and develop. Remember also that babies become very distractible around the middle of the first year, but are not ready to move completely to solid foods or cut out feedings. See Chapter 5 for discussion and help with this.

Is your child interested in solids and/or willing to take supplementation if under a year of age?

It is normal that some kids are more interested in solids than others. Solid intake can vary widely, even in the toddler years. While nursing, it is easy for your child to get most of her nutrition from your milk (with exceptions for vitamin D and iron, perhaps), and solids can be exploratory. When a child is not interested in other foods, it can be difficult to make sure that she is getting what she needs when weaned. When this is the case, many mothers take this as a sign that their child is not ready for a full weaning, and may go very slowly, partially wean, or wait altogether.

If your child is under the age of 1, it will be *absolutely necessary* to have other ways to feed her while weaning. If she isn't willing to take formula, your stored milk, or donor milk, she will not be able to get what she needs. In this situation, you may want to wait to begin weaning until she can get supplemental nutrition, or she is old enough not to need it as much.

You can encourage solid foods at any age by offering lots of healthy age-appropriate food choices. It helps to remain calm. Stress around food can have lasting effects on children, and can cause them to be more resistant rather than more open. Make sure to eat a lot of healthy foods yourself, as your child's natural interest in your food will help inspire her, and remember that there are no first foods that are as nutritionally rich as your milk, so you will want to go slowly with a younger child, nursing first, and then offering foods to make sure that she isn't too hungry when solids are offered (this can put her off of solids), and so that her health isn't impacted.

Is your child easy to redirect?

Some kids will ask to nurse but will happily do something else that is offered. Others are not going to be redirected easily, and that is okay. It is simply a sign that you need to have plans that take this into account, and that you will need to keep calm so that you don't get into power struggles.

How does your child handle change?

Just like adults, some children are naturally okay with change, and some aren't. Just like adults, children who aren't will need more preparation and patience than children who are. Parents might allow time to get used to something new *before* taking away the familiar. They can provide lots of physical reassurance and contact so that the child feels secure. They may attempt heightened sensitivity to the child's feelings and reactions, ready to reassess their plans if warranted.

An older child can be part of discussions about changes, even if still somewhat non-verbal. Ideas can be introduced and processing time given so that transitions are accepted, even with a child who has difficulty with change. You can read more about this in the sections on weaning toddlers and older children.

How does your child nurse at night?

Does he sleep for long periods or wake often? Does he nurse actively, or just suck a few times?

Children wake at night. That is part of babyhood and early childhood, and is completely normal, though there are always a few who sleep through the night from a young age and make everyone else feel like there is something wrong with their own children!

When breastfed children wake, they often want to nurse. This, too, is normal and there is nothing wrong with nursing during the night, if you continue to do so (for more on this, see Chapter 5). Remember that even an older child can be hungry during the night, especially if they are active during the day and that many children need reconnection and physical closeness if they wake at night. This is a legitimate need and will need to be factored into your plans, even if you will eventually be meeting that need in some way other than breastfeeding (Mohrbacher, 2012).

Some children will readily accept something other than nursing when they wake (cuddling, a song, rocking, water, etc.), and some will need more patience and creativity on their parents' part to do this.

Remember, if a younger baby is waking at night, feedings are still necessary and a child of this age is not capable of asking to eat when he doesn't really need to. Supplementation will be needed, so it may be a while before anyone "sleeps through the night," even without nursing.

How does your child nurse when sick or under stress?

Does she need nursing more or less during these times? Does she need to be held and comforted more, or does she run and play as usual, even with a fever? Whatever her natural tendencies are is fine; you will just want to be prepared for how you will handle them. Good plans are flexible according to need, and there are ways to change for sickness (or other stressful conditions) that won't upset all your plans.

Observing Yourself

Here are some questions you might ask as you observe yourself and your nursing relationship.

Are there nursing sessions that are particularly difficult for you?

Do you understand what is making you feel way? Would you feel better about nursing in general if a specific session or sessions were gone? Ideally, with weaning being a slow process, both you and your child will have some input on which sessions will go first, and which will be saved for last, so you may be able to drop the ones that are bothering you relatively early in the process, if they are not very important to your child. Remember, however, that feelings of resentment do not always go away because of weaning, either partially or fully. It may help you to talk with someone about your feelings as you consider weaning. Many mothers have also felt the way you do and their support may be valuable during this time.

Are there times when nursing seems sweet and enjoyable?

Again, this can help you figure out where you will begin with weaning, and what nursing sessions you will preserve until the very end.

Are there those around you who make you feel upset and worried about breastfeeding or weaning? Are there others around you who support and strengthen you?

Pressure and criticism from others can be rampant in the early years of parenting, and this is the only time in most peoples' lives when even strangers feel that they can freely criticize. This criticism may take the form of pushing weaning, or even pushing mothers *not* to wean when they feel ready to. The important thing is to find information that is good, and support that is positive and that respects your unique situation, and your expert status in your family. When you are lovingly supported, you can better give loving support to your child. If you don't have that good support in your life already, you might consider joining a mom-to-mom breastfeeding group to find it.

Are you working away from your child? How do you feel when you reconnect?

Many mothers don't realize how much easier nursing makes reconnection until it is no longer an option. Watch how you and your child reconnect, and plan for ways to continue that love and physical closeness when you are weaning.

If frustration with pumping makes you want to wean, consider whether weaning from the pump would take the pressure off, allowing you to make decisions without that as a factor. Many mothers take advantage of this and other partial-weaning options, and find that they feel much better about breastfeeding. For more information on weaning from the pump, please see Chapter 7. Mothers at La Leche League and Breastfeeding USA can also help you with ideas that they have used to wean from the pump, and for other partial weanings.

Is there a timeline you feel you need to follow?

Timelines and end-date expectations can still be compassionate if they are realistic, developmentally appropriate, and flexible enough to be reconsidered, if needed. Weaning goals can be helpful to mothers who feel best when they have plans, and they can be difficult for moms who like to wing it a bit more.

It can be helpful to consider whether you are a planner or not, and whether a timeline will be useful, or put too much pressure on you. It can also be good to ask whether you are placing an *arbitrary* timeline on yourself and your child. I have heard many mothers say they need to wean by some specific time but, with more consideration, find that there are no concrete reasons for their timeline, or that it is imposed by someone else. These mothers may still choose to begin weaning, but they won't be weaning to please others, or clinging to unrealistic ideals that, if unmet, will make them feel like they have "failed." It also means that they can relax and allow weaning to be a slow process that feels good for everyone.

Observe Your Circumstances and Family Dynamics

Here are some questions you might ask as you observe your household and the nursing relationship.

Is anything out of the ordinary happening in your family: a move, new job, divorce, sickness, etc.?

Most families find that weaning works best when no other large stressors are present, even when a baby is too young to understand them. Weaning itself can be a stressor, and if you must wean during a difficult time, your child will most likely need extra sensitivity, keen observation, and loving arms throughout the process so that he is not subject to trauma. Studies show that children have better outcomes when surrounded by loving support during stressful events (Center on the Developing Child, 2007).

What family dynamics affect your nursing relationship, specifically?

Perhaps you have an older child that needs a lot of attention, or a spouse who is worried about how long you will breastfeed. Perhaps you feel pressure from extended family, or exhaustion from older kids' activities.

Perhaps you feel uncomfortable advocating for your needs and for the needs of your nursing child, especially when it comes to weaning.

Communicating with others about the process of weaning in a positive manner is easiest if everyone understands how it works. Consider including your partner and other children in your planning so that they have realistic expectations, and feel invested and supportive. Depending on family dynamics and comfort levels regarding effective communication, some moms may also need the help of a good counselor or a book, such as *Nonviolent Communication: A Language of Life* by Marshall B. Rosenberg, PhD.

Step Three: Make a Simple, Clear, and Flexible Plan

Daunting tasks often feel much more manageable when we have a plan, even a bare-bones one. One of the best thing about having a strategy for weaning, if not on a completely child-led track, is that moms feel like they can relax and focus on one thing at a time rather than facing an amorphous void called weaning. Having specific steps to take, and working on them one at a time, builds in time that you are *not* worrying about weaning, and you and your child just get to enjoy each other. You may find that these nursings are extra sweet because they aren't tinged with any negative emotions.

After you observe your child, you can make a simple plan to follow. Your plan can be detailed, if you like, or more of an overview. It can include your thoughts and observations, ideas of how you want to begin, your goals (if applicable), and how you will handle nighttime parenting, sickness, and other situations. It can include details of how you will meet your child's needs, as well as your own and others.'

In general, all weaning plans work by eradicating feedings over time, in some fashion. This can be done by cutting them out, one at a time, whether completely or gradually. Gradual methods consist of deferring individual feedings or reducing their length. Moms have used many creative techniques to observe, explore weaning, and actively drop feedings. Here is a list of them, many of which we discuss regularly in our mom-to-mom group, and many of which I first read about in the classic weaning books, *How Weaning Happens* by Diane Bengson (1999) and *The Nursing Mother's Guide to Weaning: How to Bring Breastfeeding to a Gentle Close, and How to Decide When the Time is Right* by Kathleen Huggins and Linda Zeidrich (2007).

Practical Advice from Moms: Tips to Help You Observe and Make Your Plan

* **"Don't offer; Don't refuse" (may not be appropriate for children under 1 year of age).**

It really is just like it sounds; you aren't denying your child when she asks, and you aren't reminding her to nurse when she doesn't. Beyond being an effective observational tool for when your child really wants/needs to nurse, this is a great way to begin the weaning process without her even getting a whiff of it! It keeps things low-key for both of you, and you get to feel like you are on the journey (Bengson, 1999, p. 44).

It is important that "Don't offer; Don't refuse" is done with an open heart, and no resentment when your child *does* ask to nurse. If she feels that you are upset when she asks, anxiety may cause her to want to nurse more.

* **Get lots of "time-in."**

Children need real focused time with us to feel secure and feeling secure is how they move into new developmental stages (like weaning). Give your child lots of non-nursing cuddle time with stories and books, games, etc. If snuggling with your child makes him want to nurse, Bengson says, "Find new ways to touch your child ... : piggy-back or horsey rides, games, etc. The point is to keep that closeness, even when you aren't nursing" (Bengson, 1999, p. 47).

✳ Introduce gently.

Discuss weaning calmly as opportunities arise, when you are not trying to make anything happen. Let the concept sink in without any anxiety or anything being asked of your child (for more in-depth discussion of this gentle communication about weaning, see Chapter 1).

✳ Stand up.

Most toddlers take their mom sitting down as an invitation to nurse. That's the long and short of it. Keep standing and moving around during the day, and your toddler will most likely tend to keep himself busy.

✳ Distract and stay busy.

Moms often notice that toddlers and older nursing children don't ask to nurse much when they are out, having fun away from home. Plan playdates, take a walk, find a good park, get to know your library, or find a good place to get out in nature. If you want to be at home, invite someone over to play or plan for lots of fun art, music, and cooking projects (Bengson, 1999; Huggins & Ziedrich, 2007).

✳ Defer when possible.

Some kids just want to hear "yes," even if the things they are asking for are actually deferred. I remember being amazed when my second child would happily agree when I said, "Yes, we can nurse, but do you want to feed the dog first?" Many things that we consider chores are great fun for little ones and can help defer a nursing session. Deferring can be food-related too. Just make sure to keep it healthy so that you aren't pushing treats on your kids as a comfort substitute. When your child asks to nurse, you can say, "Sure, and I've got some strawberries (or whatever) ready to eat in the fridge! Should we go eat them?" (Bengson, 1999).

● **Keep a special set of toys or activities for when you need specific distractions.**

This can be a real lifesaver, whether you are just exploring or actively working on weaning (Bengson, 1999). These don't need to be expensive items, just ones he doesn't see often that will occupy him. Remember that your job probably won't end because you are handing him something cool instead of nursing. He may still need you to be involved and play with him. If he associates being handed a distraction with you leaving him, he may be suspicious of it next time.

● **Some good ideas for your cache of fun distractions for a toddler or older child.**

Of course, as with anything, your child may need supervision with these and you will want to make sure that your distractions are safe and not choking hazards.

- Reusable or other easy to remove stickers. Some moms even use Band-Aid™ style easy-off bandages so that kids can stick them on themselves or their mom, which is lots of fun!

- Small animals, cars, or small dolls that they haven't seen before or often

- Lift-the-flap books

- Easy art supplies and projects

- Pretend play activities

- A plastic magnifying glass and some fun things to look at

- Musical instruments or music for dancing

● **Allow nursing but end feedings a little earlier.**

Sometimes finding ways to stop nursing just a little bit earlier can really help, and can eventually lead to some sessions being dropped altogether.

There are many ways to do this and I have known a lot of moms who love this one! Bengson (1999) says,

> Some toddlers will agree to stop nursing when you count to ten, or when a timer rings, or when you have finished singing a song. Some will stop if you say, "Okay, let's play now" … Some families give these short nursings a name, such as "little bit." They allow the child little nursings during the day, and save long nursings for bedtime (p. 49).

For this method to be successful, you may not want to use it when your child really needs/expects a real nursing session (hungry, tired, etc.), at least initially (Huggins & Ziedrich, 2007).

❀ Let others help.

Weaning doesn't have to be all on you. Your child can help, if he is old enough, with the planning, and with all kinds of daily choices. Family and friends can help by providing companionship and fun when you want to limit nursing and partners, and other family members can be involved in planning and implementing.

❀ Think outside of the box.

Kids really respond to this kind of thing. You can make a little weaning book about how kids grow and change, you can have a song about nursing that helps end nursing sessions, or you can use rhymes or songs to remind kids of your proposed routine before you nurse, so they remember what they can expect.

❀ Use weaning landmarks.

If your child likes goals or making events seem special, you can plan to celebrate landmarks, such as when a child is no longer nursing during the day or during the night, or when they first choose something else when they wake up. Many families have a celebration for when their children are no longer nursing at all. The excitement of this can be a lot of fun for some kids, but again, observe carefully; some kids don't like the pressure, and some kids agree to a landmark, but don't really understand what they are agreeing to (Bengson, 1999).

❋ Allow your child to make choices.

This is one of the best ways to include your child in weaning plans. Make sure that the options you provide her are all acceptable, and that you are willing to abide by her choices. It doesn't matter whether these are big or little, which daytime nursing session to drop first, or which cup to use for nighttime water. These choices will help your child to see that her feelings are important.

❋ "Tank-up."

We are usually told not to wake a sleeping baby, so this one is new for many parents. Moms often nurse their babies to sleep (which is fine), and then go to bed themselves a few hours later, only to be waked shortly by a hungry child. This is because the child's longest stretch of sleep (perhaps 4 or 5 hours) is occurring in the first part of *their* night, and not their mom's. Many moms put off this longer stretch by waking their children gently and attempting to get a full nursing session in before their own bedtime. It may take a few days to a few weeks, but lots of moms have had success doing this, and the extra unbroken sleep makes everything about weaning (and all of parenting) easier.

❋ Keep expectations clear, and remind kids of them.

Simple words, clear expectations, and gentle reminders will keep all of you on track. Most kids need reminders *before* problems arise to be successful.

❋ Don't encourage more milk production when actively weaning.

You don't want to do things that encourage your body to make more milk during a dropped session, such as using herbs that promote milk production or fully pumping. Instead, if you feel uncomfortably full, you can pump just until you feel better (stopping here rather than fully draining your breasts), so that your body gets the message to make less.

❋ Use stock phrases and clear statements.

It really helps when everyone in the family (along with other caretakers) is using the same simple language while weaning. See what feels good to you, and try to stick to it so your child isn't confused. Make sure you are stating clearly what you *want* your child to do, not just telling her what *not* to do. For example, when you must say "no" to a nursing session, how will you do it? Rather than trying to explain every situation, it can be useful to say the same basic thing every day, such as, "We will nurse at bedtime. Let's go play _____." You can edit as needed, but you will want to keep the first part of it the same, most likely. It reminds your child of the plan. The second part tells her what you *will* do. Notice that the word "no" doesn't even need to be used.

❋ Avoid power struggles (saying "no") as much as possible.

This is never as easy as it sounds, is it? It takes practice to find ways to avoid going head-to-head with your child, and everything falls apart when you do. Learning to prevent power struggles now, while your child is young, will help you greatly as he grows. Some great resources for this are the books *Adventures in Gentle Discipline: A Parent-to-Parent Guide* by Hilary Flower, *Kids, Parents and Power Struggles* by Mary Sheedy Kurcinka, and *No-Drama Discipline: The Whole-Brain Way to Calm the Chaos and Nurture Your Child's Developing Mind* by Daniel J. Siegel and Tina Payne Bryson.

❋ Keep in mind what is developmentally normal for your child.

Breastfeeding and gentle-parenting experts know that sleep, interest in solids, independence, and other things are developmental stages that children move into when they are ready. Expect age-appropriate reactions, abilities, and behaviors from your child.

✦ Acknowledge your child's feelings.

Even if you don't understand them, their feelings are legitimate and you can accept them, help name them if they need you to, and help process them. This is another great parenting skill that will serve you for a long time to come.

I am including some sample plans mothers' stories of in each of the following sections, so that you can see some possibilities for how plans might look.

Step Four: Implement and Evaluate

Outside of unusual circumstances, try to keep to your plan for a few weeks at least, so that you can evaluate it. Remember to relax. Keep observing your child, your nursing relationship, yourself, and your family dynamics. Note what seems to work well and what doesn't. Remember that most big changes take a few days to settle in; if you can weather some strong feelings with compassion, you can make it through as long as your child is developmentally ready.

As you evaluate your plan, evaluate your feelings and desires. Have they changed? Are you feeling pressure to hurry things a bit? Are you feeling less pressure? Has your life changed? Do you need to change your weaning plan to reflect these things? Do you need more support?

If you have been working on your plan for a while and it isn't going how you had hoped, it's okay to change it, or just change the parts that aren't working. Your baby is constantly developing, and sometimes things that worked a week ago don't work anymore, and other things suddenly do. You are constantly developing as a parent (as is your partner, if you have one), and things that didn't work for you suddenly may, and vice-versa. Be open to life and its changes within the framework that you've developed.

Some moms feel that if they have implemented their plan for a while, and their child is extremely unhappy, it is a sign that they aren't developmentally ready for that part of the plan, or for the way in which it is being implemented. Be ready to do some problem solving if that occurs.

If you are afraid to change things on your plan because we are told as parents that we must always be consistent, don't worry. It is true that consistency is important, but it works best if it also occurs within a framework of love, acceptance, and flexibility. Can you be flexible and consistent at the same time? Gentle parenting advocates would say yes. In fact, being rigid isn't the same as being consistent. Consistency is a skill and rigidity is not; it is usually considered a shortcoming. Rigidity sticks to its guns, no matter what. Consistency strives to maintain a secure routine while meeting needs as they arise.

For example, if you and your partner are on a budget and never use any credit of any kind, but one of you becomes sick and the bills are more than what your savings can cover, neither of you would not consider saying, "I'm sorry you're sick, but we agreed never to take credit, so you can't have the surgery you need." Instead, you would meet the need, gladly. And certainly, you would stick to your budget in every other way, and go back to it when you could. This does not mean that you have failed in your planning. It means that you understand that, through all of life's changes, the health and well-being of every member of the family is more important than anything else.

So, there must be some loving flexibility woven into every good plan, and children need to know that their health and happiness matter. Again, this doesn't mean that we can't try to be consistent, only that we understand that rigidity in the face of clear need can tell our children that they are *not* important, and can make them feel unsafe. That is what really causes problems. If true authority is earned, we are earning it by showing that we try to make the very best decisions we can for everyone.

You may worry about how to be flexible without messing up what you have worked so hard on. Usually, communication is the key, even with a 6-to-12-month-old. Talk with your child about the situation. Talk about what you usually do, and what you are changing and why. Explain what will be expected later. They may not comprehend it all, but they understand more than we realize, and you are laying a foundation of understanding, which will remain valuable.

Here is an example: M is a 14-month-old who doesn't nurse anymore upon waking, but who is sick and asking to nurse. His mother says, "Poor sweetie, I know you feel so bad. You want to nurse. We don't nurse when we wake up anymore. We go play! Do you want to go play with your trains? No? Do you want ride in the stroller? Do you want to feed the cat? You still need to nurse? Okay, Mama will nurse because you are *so* sick. But tomorrow, when you are feeling better, we will play when you wake up."

Usually, children go back to their regular habits when they feel better. They want to be active and play again and, even if they ask to nurse, will be easy to distract if they were before. We can help by reminding them of the regular routine when they feel better: "You are feeling so much better. I'm so glad! When we wake up in the morning, we are going to jump up, and eat some banana and cereal, and go to the park to play," and then when morning comes, we keep our word. We have the bananas and cereal ready, and the stroller too.

There will come a time when you may *not* feel it is appropriate to go back to nursing, even when your child is sick, or under some other stress, but if you are still on the weaning journey, you can use your own instincts.

What if your partner isn't comfortable with observing and changing your plan?

Check to see that the plan isn't just *your* plan (or yours and your baby's), and not a team plan that meets your partner's needs too. Offer a non-judgmental ear, really try to listen to what worries and hopes are being expressed, and remember that most of us grew up with parents who were told never to give in or change their rules for fear of losing their authority. This may be a real fear for your partner. See if your partner has some reasonable ideas for your plan, and if there are compromises that the two of you can make without compromising the security and needs of your child.

Another part of evaluating is remaining calm and not allowing small setbacks to upset you. Setbacks of many kinds will happen all through your life, and your child's life. Staying in the moment, and acknowledging the things that you cannot change with graceful acceptance teaches your children how to manage their own setbacks.

It can be easy and even fun, sometimes, to plan. It can be a lot harder to implement it, especially when you are tired or overwhelmed, so be prepared that implementation may take some commitment! If your child has a "more passionate" nature than yours, you may find it difficult to stick with your plans when things are hard and your child has strong feelings. The books mentioned in the "Avoid Power Struggles" tip earlier in Step Three may help you with this.

When something in the plan doesn't feel good or seems very difficult, it is important to try to figure out what the problem is *before* you make changes. Usually, the way to figure out what is going on is to wait until you have a quiet moment and you are a few hours past the difficulty. Give yourself a chance to think: What happened beforehand? Was your child prepared? Were you too tired or busy to implement things the way you had planned? Did you jump to anger or worry quickly? Was there an unusual stressor, such as pain, exhaustion, work pressures, etc.? Has your child told you that they don't feel comfortable with this area of your plan, either in words or actions? Do you feel comfortable with this aspect of your plan?

Through calm evaluation of your plan, you may be able to see that your plan needs to change, or that behavior/stressors need to be modified. If you feel you may have dropped the ball a bit, or been operating in automatic mode rather than a thinking mode, you can forgive yourself and try again next time. That's the cool thing about kids; you get to try again!

Depending on the age of your child, you may be able to ask them what didn't work, or what could be done better. Even young children can surprise us with great ideas, and they always enjoy being listened to and taken seriously.

If you decide to change your plan, make it clear to everyone. Write it on your plan. Tell your child, and tell your partner or other caregivers. Be proud of your ability to problem-solve and test out this new aspect of your plan.

Sometimes, children experience temporary periods of regression. It may be impossible to know why a child's needs temporarily change, but it happens fairly frequently and it isn't the child's fault. This time will pass and, with a baby, usually all that is required is patience and willingness to meet his needs. With an older child, you can have a dialogue to figure out what is happening, and what can be done. Again, your plans won't be completely torn apart if you meet your child's needs differently for a day or two as long as you discuss it with him! I remember once my daughter, who hadn't nursed during the night for over a week, had some bug bites on her ankle and was so itchy that she couldn't sleep. She was crying and tossing around, and begging to nurse. I said, "We will nurse in the morning," my stock phrase, over and over, but it just wasn't working. I finally nursed her, telling her it was only because of the bug bites, and she quickly fell asleep. The next night, she asked again and I said, "Remember, that was only because of your bug bites. We will nurse in the morning." She looked at me for a minute, and then turned over and let me put her to bed.

As you evaluate, make sure to reflect on the good work you are all doing. Kids love to talk about the things that they can do and, like anyone else, they like to hear that they are working hard and doing a good job. Also, because many of us tend to focus on what isn't done, yet instead of what is going well, it can be nice to remind yourself that you are making progress, no matter how slow.

CHAPTER 9

Weaning Plans for Different Ages

Creating a Weaning Plan for a Child from 6 Months to 1 Year of Age

There may be something going on in your life that makes nursing for the recommended duration impossible, especially if you do not have the support that you need to continue. You are the expert on your family, and the decision of whether you need to wean is yours. If you are being told that you *must* wean, but would like to know if this is true, please see Chapter 2 for a discussion of "Unexpected and Serious Circumstances," and the chapters in Section Two for Frequently Asked Questions that may address your situation.

Nursing, even for 6 months, is so much more than many mothers are willing to do. I hope that you feel great pride in this accomplishment. The benefits that you have given to your child are huge. You are a loving mother, and your strong bond will continue as you wean and beyond. Even at this age, you will be able to be compassionate and keep your connection with your baby strong.

Three Things to Remember When Weaning a Baby Under the Age of 1

1. A child this age will need supplementation of some sort as you cut breastfeeding sessions, even if eating solids.
2. You will want to *proceed slowly,* as abrupt weaning is rarely recommended, and because you and your child are more vulnerable to possible complications at this age. Your baby and your body need time to adjust; the last thing you'll want to deal with as you wean is mastitis!
3. A baby still has powerful physical and emotional need for you, whether or not she is nursing. Some moms find themselves distancing themselves when no longer nursing, and this can be traumatic for babies.

Note: I am not including anything in this book for weaning before the age of 6 months because a child younger than 6 months of age will require consultation with a doctor to make sure that her needs are met.

Step One: Relax

Again, most likely you do not have to make some big change *today.* You have the time to breathe and to think about how you want to do this and how it will work for your family and your child. If your child has tasted solids, you are already on the road to weaning.

Many babies between 6 months and 1 year of age are still nursing very regularly, even when eating solids, and they really love nursing. That's a big reason why parents try to be compassionate when working on weaning. Your child is at an age where you cannot easily discuss your plans with them, so your physical and emotional availability is very important; she needs this to stay connected with you.

So, breathe, relax if you can, hold your child, and try to enjoy some of the sweetness of nursing her before you move into your plan. You will feel more able to plan and think clearly if you are not under stress.

Step Two: Observe

Observation is the primary way that a planned weaning under the age of 1 can be a partnership between a mother and baby. This is how you show your child kindness, and take her needs into account. You will never regret this loving approach, and you will be rewarded for it as your bond remains strong, even as your breastfeeding relationship winds down.

During this observation period, you are simply evaluating your child's needs, so that you are not jumping in with a rigid plan that won't work for anyone. You are assessing your own feelings, needs, and the present situation in your household.

The observation questions and tips in Chapter 8 may help you get a sense of how your particular breastfeeding relationship works. These observations about you and your child and your family will help you create the right plan for your needs.

Step Three: Make a Simple, Clear, and Flexible Plan

Remember that when weaning at this time, your body will be more impacted than if your child was older. If you cut out a feeding, experts Nancy Mohrbacher and Kathleen Kendall-Tackett recommend taking several days to get used to this change before you consider cutting another. You can "pump just to comfort" (stopping as soon as you feel relief, rather than pumping fully), or hand express (also "just to comfort") if needed (2010, p. 173).

Try to keep your weaning expectations realistic for your baby. She is still quite young and at a vulnerable age. She can only do what she can do; she is a creature of instinct, unable to manipulate or want anything she doesn't truly need. You, however, can evaluate and change as circumstances dictate, and you can be understanding about her needs, even as you begin to meet them in a different manner.

An Example of Observations and a Simple Plan for a Baby

Observations (By the Mother)

Nighttime: Jay (6 months old) usually wakes two or three times during the night. Sometimes he will nurse a lot, but other times he just sucks a few times and falls asleep. He usually starts the night in his crib in our room, but ends up in our bed when he wakes. We are okay with this for now, but hope that when he is weaned, he will stay in the crib. Jay only wants me to put him to bed and goes to sleep nursing.

Waking: Jay nurses quickly, but heavily, when he first wakes, and then wants to get out of bed to find his older brothers.

Daytime: He is on the go after waking for three or four hours, maybe nursing once, then he nurses to sleep for his nap around 1:00. When he wakes, he nurses again for a few minutes, and plays until supper. He nurses once or twice between his nap and bedtime.

Personality: I think Jay has a strong will, and he gets very upset when he can't have something he wants. However, he is also easily distracted, and feels better if his brothers play with him or something. Jay can be comforted by his brothers and Dad, as well as me, but not by anyone outside the family.

Solids: Liking them so far! Has tasted avocado and sweet potato.

Sickness: Jay doesn't sleep as much when he is sick. He nurses a lot when he is sick, and doesn't want to do anything except be held.

Me: I am nervous about weaning because extended family members and friends constantly ask when we will wean. I don't feel comfortable talking about it, and feel like I have to listen to my mother and grandmother's advice.

I am going back to work when the next school year starts in 3 months. The hours are long and begin very early, so I feel like weaning needs to happen soon. Jay will be at a good daycare.

I worry especially about nursing first thing in the morning because I have to wake very early and get Jay to daycare. My husband will be helping my other boys get to school.

I enjoy bedtime nursing most because I can rest and relax. I do not feel worried because it helps me get sleepy too.

I do worry about nursing to sleep for naps though, because he will be at daycare during that time. I feel like he needs other ways to get to sleep. I have tried rocking, patting, and walking while his dad tried on weekends, but it has not worked so far.

I feel concerned about nighttime nursing, because I need to get enough sleep to do my job. I don't feel too worried *while* nursing during the night, but when I think about it later, I get worried.

I feel ready to wean so that I can focus on my job, as well as my family. I know that other teachers have worked and nursed, but Jay will be 9 months old, and I don't feel like I can handle both. I have talked with several people, and I feel okay with my decision, and I expect it to take a few months.

My husband is happy to leave this decision to me and doesn't seem worried about it.

My Plan for Jay's Weaning

1. I will wait for 2 weeks to begin. I will relax and give myself permission to enjoy nursing without worrying about anything!
2. We'll protect bedtime nursing until last and keep enjoying it. The same goes for nighttime nursing. I won't worry about it for now, and we'll let it go next to last.
3. We'll work first on daytime, making sure to be active and have lots of distractions. I'll drop one daytime nursing at a time, slowly. I feel that this is the easiest time to begin, but I'll nurse for now if he is sick, and worry about what to do about that later. I will make sure to have a bottle of formula and some snacks ready at all times.

4. Next, we'll work on waking. I'll wake up first, and have toys and a bottle ready by the bed, in case he wakes before the big kids. If I am sleeping in on the weekend, Dad will be ready to help. Naps will look the same: toys and food ready and something exciting to do. Maybe we'll have a stroller ready to walk to the park.

5. Nighttime nursing next. I'll have a sippy cup of water ready, and a Yoga Ball to bounce him. If he goes right back to sleep, he will go into crib. If he needs more, I will give him a bottle. I will see how this goes and change strategy, if I need to.

6. Last is naptime and bedtime. We'll begin a bedtime routine with a bath (at night), maybe a book (may not work as he is so active), rocking in chair or bouncing on yoga ball, singing, rubbing back or patting, *then* nursing. I want to try to get him used to other things before removing nursing. Maybe he will fall asleep while rocking or bouncing. I like doing this, and don't mind continuing after weaning.

7. Timeline: Baby Jay will be weaned, except maybe for bedtime (not sure about this, yet), by the time next school year starts.

8. Tidbits: I will try not to worry about what we haven't gotten to! We'll just enjoy each other. I will hold Jay even when I won't nurse him so that he knows I love him. I will tell daycare workers that I want him held if he is crying.

Step 4: Implement and Evaluate

As you implement your plan and evaluate what works and what doesn't, remember that it can be much more difficult to understand what is happening with a child younger than one than it might be with an older child. Because they often lack speech, our understanding of babies' feelings is subject to our translation of their sounds, facial expressions and movements, as is the perceived reasons for these feelings. Remember that your baby is a complete human being unto himself with a different personality and different reactions than you have. Try to observe him without ascribing him assumed or negative motivations. He is not trying to manipulate you or your situation – he is still a creature of pure instincts, communicating his needs however he can. Even when you cannot meet these needs in the ways he would like best, this understanding can prevent anger and frustration and can keep you responsive and kind throughout this sensitive time.

If something isn't working, consider whether what you are asking of your child is developmentally appropriate and whether it can be changed a bit. Consider whether it is necessary at the moment, or can be left for a bit later. For example, if you came up with a morning routine that would have you both getting up and eating instead of nursing but your baby is very unhappy with this and not moving past it, even after a week or two, consider what might change that you can both live with. Is it possible that he misses not only the nursing but also the closeness, the sweet morning snuggling? Could you sit together somewhere and do this, really connecting, before you eat? Could you consider working on this nursing session last, focusing instead on removing the ones that seem less important to him? Remember, as we discussed in Chapter 8, you aren't undermining your authority by revamping your plan, rather you are showing your child that you can listen and that his feelings are important to you.

So, how did Baby's Jay's plan work?

His mom says: "Well, we got all of the weaning plan done easily except it was very hard to get Jay to sleep for his nap without nursing. I did not get this figured out before going back to work. Also, I decided not to cut bedtime because I enjoyed it and didn't really see the point.

I was worried about naptime at daycare, but he ended up playing until he fell asleep in the teacher's arms most of the time. Rocking worked for them (never for me) if they did it as soon as he seemed sleepy.

At home on the weekends, I still nurse him to sleep for his nap and for bedtime. Honestly, I kind of like it. I have always had a hard time falling asleep, and nursing before bed calms me down. We have decided to keep doing this for a while. We don't nurse during the night. He was mad the first few nights, but I rocked him and sang to him, and eventually, he got used to taking a bottle of formula and cuddling.

Mostly, the plan worked great! When he had the flu, I nursed him several times in the day and night even though we had been down to just bedtime and naptime. Later, he didn't actually seem to remember that he had been nursing again. I think because he was pretty out of it."

Here Are Some More Moms' Stories

Anonymous

I began weaning my daughter at 6 months because I had postpartum depression. I really feel like nursing made it harder for me because I felt worse when I had to sit or lie still, like I was being smothered. If I was up and doing things, I felt a little better.

I saw a therapist when my friend suggested I might have PPD. She helped, but I still felt terrible when I was nursing. My boyfriend and I talked it over and decided that if I weaned, he could help more with feeding, and I could feed her while I was standing up. I felt good about the decision and was going to do it cold turkey when the same friend talked with me about doing it a little more slowly to make sure I didn't get mastitis.

I started replacing nursing with a bottle of pumped milk once a day. She took the bottle well. I hand expressed a little milk into the sink when I felt full. She was only nursing once during the night, so I started having my boyfriend feed her then. The only problem was that I was still awake and jittery when he was helping her. I still felt smothered just lying in bed, so I had to get up and walk around until I was calm.

I had her down to two breastfeedings a day (formula and solids the rest of the time after my pumped milk was gone), and I was still feeling bad. My daughter seemed to be doing fine, though, and I was with her all day, so I stood up with her and danced around, and played on the floor with her as much as I could. I ended up taking an antidepressant, and when I did, I went ahead and weaned completely because the doctor said I should. I think now moms are told that they can keep nursing. I started feeling better pretty quickly.

I did the best I could. As bad as I felt, totally not like myself, I am amazed that I took care of her and nursed at all! My daughter is 5 now, and we have a lot of fun together. I don't have to take medication, and we are very close and have fun together. I had planned for nursing to be different and I was shocked with how it really was for me. But I know this; love conquers all!

Nicole O.

Let me start by saying that I wanted to do everything right when it came to pregnancy, breastfeeding, and childrearing. I read books, talked to older female relatives, and did research on the internet. Years later, looking back on how it all went, I did do it right: right for me. Sure, I've learned some things over the years, and I probably could have done some things differently, but we can only do our best with what we know.

My son was born in the spring of 2000, and I was 24 years old. I couldn't get him to latch on for about the first 8 hours after birth, and the nurse was getting more and more insistent that we feed him a bottle of formula. I had read that doing so could interfere with the process, so I resisted. Finally, after one more try, he latched on and gulped greedily, sputtering because the flow was so fast and he wasn't used to eating yet.

Nursing went well, for the most part, after I learned how to hold him properly. I really enjoyed lying on the couch with him, watching his eyes droop tiredly after his tummy started getting full. I decided to wean at about 6 months. I really had no idea how long people could or should nurse, but I felt like I wanted to have more freedom of movement. I slowly transitioned him to bottles over the course of a month or two. I still gave him a nighttime feeding for some time. It went pretty smoothly as far as I remember, and he has always been a good eater. I think part of the reason I decided to wean at that age is because nursing in public was difficult for me, and not really accepted at that time. I was still in college, and enough people stared at me already for bringing a baby on campus.

127

Laura G.

When my first son was 8 months old, I started feeling extremely tired, and joked that the last time I was this tired, I was pregnant—and it turned out that I was. I went to the doctor for my first prenatal visit and asked if I should continue to breastfeed. I think a big part of me wanted him to say, "no," but he said "of course." I was tired, and a little overwhelmed at the thought of two babies so close together. My son was eating solids by this time, and preferred them. He only nursed before going to sleep and in the middle of the night. There was this big part of me that wanted to continue to nurse him. I still enjoyed and loved that I could help him go to sleep and comfort him, and another part that was just tired. In the end, however, he was fully weaned at about 10 months. I was 4 months pregnant at that point. The transition was very smooth and gradual for both of us, and I was glad to know that I could still comfort him and be close to him.

Creating a Weaning Plan for a Child Who is Between 1 and 2 Years of Age

You've made it to the recommended minimum for breastfeeding and perhaps beyond. Maybe, in the beginning, you couldn't imagine being able to do it this long and, now, here you are. Maybe now it is difficult for you to imagine *not* doing it, but you are feeling like you and your child might be ready to wean.

Remember that this decision is yours, your child's, and your partner's (if you have one), and no one else's. Other people may have especially aggressive opinions about breastfeeding as your child passes the age of 1 but there are many benefits you still provide to your child and to yourself when you breastfeed beyond 1 year (for a list of some, please see Chapter 6) and most other people are completely unaware of them. If you are enjoying your breastfeeding relationship, but are feeling pressure from outside to wean, you may want to seek support before you decide to begin weaning in earnest.

You probably know by now that the process of weaning begins when your child first samples solids. Even if your child does not enjoy large amounts of solid food (which is normal for some children), and still nurses quite often, you are on the road to weaning. This can be very helpful for moms to remember if they are feeling worried about the weaning process. You and your child have probably already begun.

Step One: Relax

Take a bit of time, if you can, to enjoy this phase of your life and connect with your child. She will never be this age again, and your relationship will never be quite this symbiotic again. Even if you are ready to quit, taking a bit of time to relax will help you see your situation with clear eyes and a calm mind.

Step Two: Observe

This second step can be relaxed too. Your job is to observe your child, yourself, your relationship, your family, and your life. No judgement, just observation. Each component of your breastfeeding situation is important and will be part of the best plan for *your* life and *your* family. Read the observation questions in the previous chapter of this book, and note what you see and feel. This observation is one of the easiest ways to partner with your child. Remember that you are the expert, and your observations are the ones that truly come from a place of understanding and love.

Don't worry that some nursing sessions may look like they are more about comfort than food (and nursing does much more than just these two things, anyway). Comfort is a legitimate need for your child and, indeed, for all humans. Being able to comfort your child is a beautiful thing, and mothers of nursing toddlers highly prize this aspect of nursing, and often describe it as a reset button. For more discussion on comfort, see the Frequently Asked Questions in Chapter 6.

Step Three: Make a Simple, Clear, and Flexible Plan

One of the most exciting things about weaning children over age 1 is that you can talk with them about it. The idea isn't to stress them out, threatening to take this lovely thing away from them, but you can slowly introduce the idea of weaning, and give them some choices in how it is carried out.

Use your observations, goals, and the tips in the Practical Advice from Moms section in the previous chapter to make your plan. Invite input from everyone in your family, and keep your plans realistic, age-appropriate, kind, and flexible. Make sure your plan includes simple, easy-to-follow steps with ideas for what to do in special situations.

An Example of Observations and a Simple Plan for a Toddler

Observations and Plans Run Together in This One and Are Written by Mom

Stella (18 mos.) only wants me, most of the time. Even Dad can have a hard time when she is upset. I am due in 5 months with baby #2. I'm not totally against tandem nursing, but I'm really hoping that Stella can be weaned before the baby comes.

Habits: Stella has three "noosies" that she never misses, no matter what. She nurses when she wakes up in the morning, or from her nap, for a long time. It's like she needs to get courage and comfort before facing the day. She usually falls asleep for her nap on her own. She plays on the floor, and then eventually crawls onto the couch with her blanket and falls asleep. I tried offering some little toys when she woke from her nap a couple of times, just to see what would happen. She turned her head from them and started to fuss. Twenty minutes or so of nursing, and she is ready to play.

Bedtime: After dinner, we have started a long bedtime routine including a bath, teeth brushing, books, baby massage, setting up a sippy cup of water, tucking in a stuffed animal with her, and a song. Then we nurse until she turns over to sleep (10 or 15 minutes). When Dad tried to do bedtime things with her, she cried and needed me. We want to change that before the baby comes.

Nighttime: I am so tired with this pregnancy, and I want Stella to either sleep all night, or let her dad help her. After some research and discussion with other moms, I know that Stella may not be ready to sleep straight through yet, and I like that she doesn't usually want to nurse very much during the night. She usually wakes up (in her little bed in our room) and cries. I go and talk to her and pat her back. Sometimes she won't settle and needs to nurse (we notice this happens most when the day has been stressful, or she didn't get a long-enough nap, so we'll work on those things too), but most of the time, she settles quickly, and goes back to sleep and doesn't wake again until about 6 a.m. Our plan is to have her dad work with her during the night. If she settles, fine. If she needs nursing (for the moment), that is fine too. We will have a cup of water by the bed and her glow-turtle, and Dad will attempt to help her back to sleep without nursing, if possible. We will remind her at bedtime about not nursing during the night. We're going to observe this a bit more with Dad helping to see if we can just take this one out. I think we can, but we want to watch what happens first. We will revisit. Nighttime will probably be our second planned time of "no."

Daytime: How much Stella nurses during the day depends on what we are doing. At home, it can be often. When we are out, she only asks if she is hurt or tired. After nursing in the morning and having breakfast, we will keep a busy schedule until naptime. I will remember to do some physical things to help wear Stella out. We will walk to the swimming pool or playground every day, and meet friends at these places, if we can. We will pack a picnic lunch to stay out longer. We will get Stella some cool, big-girl things to take with her and/or use at home: a backpack, water bottles and cups, picnic plates, and utensils. When we come home, I will put out her books and blocks, and let her play until she is ready to sleep, as usual. When she wakes, I will nurse her, while quietly talking about things we can do. I want to begin to associate waking up with something fun, and we'll try watering the plants first, because she loves that. I think, at some point, we will be able to just do that when she wakes.

Dad likes to connect with Stella when he comes home, but he also likes to cook dinner. I am usually beat by that time, so it is hard to be active, and Stella tends to sit around with me, nursing while Dad cooks. But if there is something more interesting going on, she will do that instead. This is going to be our first "no" to nursing, but we are going to try very hard not to make it feel like "no." We have agreed that we would feel okay about Stella watching an educational show while Dad cooks in the evenings. Before the show, I will remind Stella that she can watch a show instead of nursing. If she is upset, I will distract her. I'll take her outside to swing, or Dad will have her help him cook.

Food: Stella doesn't eat a lot, but she likes to sit with us at dinner, and play and eat a bit. We noticed she eats more when she helps Dad cook, so we will try to do this more often. We will try to offer more snacks during the day too.

Special situations: Stella takes after me a bit. We both get easily thrown off by life events and need some time to get back on track. Watching the last few weeks, I realize that I don't do much preparation with her. I think I was so used to her as a baby, just happy to be snuggled up with me wherever or whatever was happening, that I didn't get that she was older now and trying to make sense of things. She needs me to tell her what's happening, and why, and she seems to understand quite a bit of it. It's funny, I always sort of made fun of moms who explain everything to their 1-year-old. But it really helps! So, I am going to talk with her about changes and things we expect. Thinking of how she handles stress, we decided that if she is upset when we can't nurse, we'll hold her and comfort her through it. We won't expect her to be a different kid. We'll try to distract and say "no" as gently as we can.

When the baby comes, and she is totally or mostly weaned, she might want to nurse again. If she asks, we have decided to keep that as a "no." I don't want to start again if she has finished. If she is still nursing a bit, we will remind her of the times she can nurse, and keep to them only. Dad will be in charge of this, and we will try to involve her in the baby's nursing as much as possible (getting diapers ready, bringing mom water, rubbing the baby's back).

Introducing: We are making a book together (me and Stella) about Big Kids Weaning (author's note: If you decide to use words like "big kid," be careful that this never moves into shaming. Make sure that your child never feels bad about the times that they can't act like a big kid, and are not told they are "acting like a baby," etc.; Edson, 2016). Grandma is going to get her a soft doll that isn't a baby. We will show her baby doll nursing and the other doll eating food. We will do anything else we can do to introduce the topic in a relaxed way, without pushing too much.

Ending: We are thinking about doing some sort of "big sister" day when we do our baby shower. Maybe we'll celebrate weaning too, if we can get there. We are waiting a bit to introduce the idea so she doesn't have to wait too long and so we can see how it is going.

Step Four: Implement and Evaluate

Implementation and Evaluation are the active aspects of your overall weaning plan and the only way to know if it is a good weaning plan is to commit to it for a while, to see what works and what doesn't. The exception to this is when any part of your plan is quickly evident as disrespectful or hurtful to anyone involved. As time goes on, it will become clear what changes are needed, if any.

As I mentioned in the discussion of this step in Chapter 8, you don't have to be afraid that change will undermine your authority, as long as you explain to your toddler what is happening in simple, age-appropriate terms. For example, "I think we need to go back to nursing when we wake up, just until you are a little bigger. We have tried for so long and you are still so sad all day, even at daycare. How about I sing one song to you while we nurse in the morning and then..." Involve your child as much as you can in the change, either with her ideas and choices, or with your knowledge of what she likes to do that could be a good transition: fresh strawberries each morning after nursing for one song, having a picnic breakfast outside after a quick nursing, etc.

So, how did Stella's plan go?

It took 4 months for Stella to fully wean.

In carrying out Stella's plan above, her mom and dad noticed a few things. First of all, Stella handled the evening changes amazingly well. She began with watching an educational show, but now she often prefers to pull up a chair and help her dad cook. Her mom has been going out into the yard and relaxing by herself during this time. Once, when Stella got hurt, her mom came inside to help and Stella wanted to nurse. Mom said that they would nurse at bedtime and stuck with it, walking with her, holding her, and singing to her. Eventually, Stella calmed down, but wanted to be held. Mom and Dad knew it was important that Stella felt loved *and* that they tried to stick with their plan to see if it was working. Mom decided to keep holding her and walked around outside with her until dinner was ready. It worked and she accepted not nursing at that time.

What *didn't* work well was their nighttime plan. When Dad helped Stella, they found that she asked for nursing more often than she usually did. Dad tried to distract her, but then Mom nursed if Stella seemed to really need it. As a result, Mom was getting less sleep than before. They decided that they needed to change their plan. They felt they were confusing Stella, and needed to consistently say "no" or "yes," and not go back and forth. They decided that they didn't want to nurse until the morning, and that they were willing to help her accept this, even if it meant a few hard nights at first. Dad wanted to take this over so Mom could sleep. He made a new picture book about Stella's nighttime.

He showed Mom dreaming and growing the baby. In the dream, she was thinking about Stella and holding her, which was a great touch. The picture book showed the things Stella *could* do at night, and showed Stella nursing again when she woke up, the sun was shining, and Mom was ready. They decided to implement this plan immediately by reading the book, preparing her for it for a few days, and then doing it. Stella loved the book, but when the first night came, she was very anxious and cried a lot. Dad stayed with her and reminded her of what they were doing. The next week varied: sometimes difficult, sometimes easy. She is happier now when she wakes, and doesn't ask to nurse. She asks for her dad and her book.

More Mothers' Stories

Anonymous

When my son was 16 months old, he was nursing all the time, day and night. I wasn't enjoying nursing much anymore, though I had when he was a baby. None of the moms close to me were still nursing a kid this old, and I felt embarrassed a bit.

My neighbor nursed all four kids, and I went over to her house with my son to talk with her. I sat down on her couch, and my son immediately started pulling my shirt up to nurse. Even though I knew she was breastfeeding friendly, I felt embarrassed and tried to distract him. She said it was fine to nurse, so I did. He sat there nursing the whole time we were there. Like, for 45 minutes!

I told my neighbor how I felt. She gave me a book about breastfeeding toddlers. She said she had breastfed her last child until he was 3 and a half, and that she didn't see anything wrong with it. She said she would have done it longer, but he stopped.

The book was good, but I still had a problem. I realized that there was nothing wrong with continuing to nurse, and that there were benefits. I knew that I would be happy to continue, even if I felt embarrassed, if he wasn't nursing so constantly and for so long! My neighbor connected me with some other moms she knew who had nursed toddlers, and they gave me some tips. One mom showed me a sign she had made that said: "Do new things! Get out of your comfort zone!" She said she put it on her fridge, and ended up cutting out daytime nursing almost completely by getting out and doing things. Another mom mentioned that my son was meeting some sort of need by nursing so much. She said that I should keep it in mind because there was something going on: a need I would still have to help him with.

Honestly, now I think he was bored. I am not a very active person, and I enjoy staying at home and relaxing with my son, who used to just play happily around the house. I preferred it to working outside the house, which was why I changed to working part-time from home after maternity leave. But he was older now, and I hadn't figured out anything new for him to do.

I started working when he was sleeping and started doing other things during the day. I joined a playgroup, which was hard for me to do, but it was great. My son loved it and I started to see that he is different than I am. He really needs social time, and I could take it or leave it. We started going to the park every day, and the library if it rained. We packed food and were out of the house just after breakfast, all the way to afternoon nap. After that, we did chores around the house and played together. Within a month, we weren't nursing during the day at all!

Nighttime was different. He was still nursing. I'm not sure how many times, but it was at least three or four. I was okay with night nursing for a while. That really surprised me! I think once I got rid of the anger at him for nursing all the time, and when I nursed less during the day, I was fine. We night-weaned about 6 months later when I decided to go back to work full-time. It was partly his idea because he said he wanted a racecar bed like his friend had. He said he didn't need me to sleep with him because he was big. I thought he would wake and nurse, at least at first, but he didn't. He was down to only nursing at bedtime after that, and we did that for another month.

Honestly, none of it was that hard, and we just kept acting like we always did, talking about everything and being together. The hard parts were understanding what was going on, and changing my way of doing things.

Ann

I am a planner. Absolutely. I can't stand to do anything without a plan. I had a plan for birth. I had a plan for initiating breastfeeding. And I had a plan for maternity leave. But I had not considered weaning.

Our daughter was just over 1 year old when my husband asked, "So, what's the weaning plan?" and was shocked that I didn't have one. So, off I went to plan! I researched, talked with moms at La Leche League, read blogs, and I came back with a plan. My husband said, "This will take months! I thought we could just do it." I was shocked. He didn't usually have opinions about this kind of thing. I finally got it out of him: he had noticed people giving us looks in church when we nursed and it made him uncomfortable.

I revised my plan to include not nursing in the service at church. That was the first thing. It wasn't too hard. I just sat in the nursery with her (she wasn't ready to stay by herself) and played. If she wanted to nurse, I went walking with her around the church instead, or got her a snack.

I hadn't nursed her to sleep since she was about 8 months old. I had decided to nurse her, and then rub her back in her crib, and we were still doing that, though we never did any cry-it-out. However, she was still waking to nurse during the night a few times. My plan was to night wean completely next. I think she was a little young, maybe, because she was still very hungry. She would wake once or twice, and go back to sleep, but every night at about 4 in the morning, she wouldn't go back to sleep, no matter what we did. She kept signing "milk!" My husband said that maybe the plan needed some tweaking, and I got a bit mad because I liked my plan! But the next day, I thought about it and realized that it did need changing. I decided to skip that step for just that one nighttime nursing, and moved on to daytime stuff.

Daytime was easier. I did the "don't offer; don't refuse" thing, and saw that she only seemed to care about nursing when she woke up, and when she got hungry or tired. We started having her favorite foods for breakfast, and nursing for shorter and shorter times in the morning by counting to 10 at the end. Soon, we were only doing it for 10 seconds! Then we started using the 10 seconds for everything.

At 18 months, she was nursing once during the night and twice during the day (daytime was counting slowly to 10). Amazingly, she could get milk in 10 seconds! At 20 months, she was only nursing once at night. Just before her second birthday, we dropped the night nursing. She cried every night for almost a week, but I stuck with it and stayed with her, rubbing her back, holding her, and giving her water. She would only let me do it, not her dad.

So, my plan didn't work perfectly. The process helped me figure out that I couldn't make plans that affected my family without their input! I still love to plan. I can't help it! But I always ask if they are okay with my plans.

Creating a Weaning Plan for a Child Who is Over 2 Years of Age

There can be some truly beautiful partnership when weaning older children. They can be included to a much greater degree than younger children and, of course, their ability to do this only increases as they grow. It can be a lot of fun to plan with them because they can look toward future goals, such as weaning celebrations or other special markers of their progress. They can understand what is being asked of them and make informed choices when allowed.

This is a time of growth spurts for mothers, not just for children. As our babies turn into bigger kids, we can feel some normal desires to start meeting our own needs, and we can feel frustrated with breastfeeding and other small-child needs that are still present. The good news is that we can learn to meet our own needs and to communicate effectively about them *while* being compassionate with weaning.

You and your child may end up with an unscheduled, child-led weaning, or you may take specific steps to partially or fully wean. You may work on this over the course of a few months, or a year or two. It's up to you, your child, and your family. The steps are the same as for a younger child.

Step One: Relax

Once again, nothing must happen this second, and there is great benefit in stepping back, breathing, and relaxing. Good observation and planning are going to happen when your mind is receptive, and you are not working under worried or hurried conditions. So, give yourself a break. Close your eyes and breathe. This is going to happen, no matter what, and you are going to help it happen with love.

Step Two: Observation

The next step is observation. It is an enjoyable step because it requires you to do nothing but watch. Yet, it is getting you somewhere, and giving you some time to just be with your child, to experience the sunset of this sweet time with him, instead of missing it by being preoccupied with worry or plans.

There are a lot of facets to the breastfeeding relationship, even with an older child. Your job, for now, is to look at all of them with as objective an eye as you are able. Every part of your life together is important, and this honest look is integral to creating a good weaning plan, even if your plan is to let him wean in an unscheduled, child-led manner (because what if your child loves plans and schedules, and you need to be open to that?). Take a bit of time to just watch everything with no judgements, noting things as you see them. You can use the observation questions in Chapter 8 as a starting place, if you need one.

Step Three: Make a Simple, Clear, and Flexible Plan

As you create your plan, you can be as general or specific as you'd like and as long it is clear and simple enough for your whole family to follow, it won't matter exactly what it looks like. The nice thing, as I have said, about weaning plans for older kids is that they can be really involved and invested, so make sure to invite input from everyone! The tips and techniques that other mothers have used to explore and encourage weaning may be of great value to you with a child over the age of two, so please feel free to read about them in the Practical Advice from Moms section in the last chapter.

An Example of Observations and a Simple Plan for an Older Child

(This weaning plan is for Joe, 2 ½ years old, written by his mom.)

Observations

General: Nursing is quick. Joe jumps in my lap and nurses for 4 or 5 minutes. Joe is easy to distract, but I am usually so tired that I'd rather nurse him and play on my phone, or read a book, than figure out something else to do. I am going to be more active. I realized I sit all the time when I am home! I am going to try to stand up as much as I can because I really think that he is triggered to nurse when I sit! Wow, I hadn't realized that.

Sleep: Joe nurses to sleep if I am home, both napping and bed. He falls asleep quickly, and once he is out, I can leave him in the bed. He sleeps in my bed, and I am okay with that, until he is ready for a big bed in my room. He only wakes once during the night unless something is wrong. I haven't offered anything else during the night yet, but we have been talking about it a little (how he won't always need to, and what other things kids do in the night). When I am working an evening shift, he reads with Sara (his much older sister) to fall asleep, and drinks water in a sippy cup.

Eating: Joe has gotten more interested in food in the last few months.

We have replaced all pumped milk when I am gone with food (yay, no more pumping!).

Comfort: Joe is the easiest kid in the world when everything is good, but when it isn't, he is hard to comfort without nursing. Sara is better at this than I am because she can usually make him laugh. When I am alone, it always seems easier to nurse him. Also, I am not great at playing the way Sara is, and I get easily overwhelmed with the noise, especially if I have been working. I want to figure out how to comfort him in other ways, but I am anxious about that.

Me/Family Dynamic: I am very nervous about weaning! I feel like I understand nursing, and it is so easy, but he is getting older, and I am working more (and an ER nurse's hours are all over the place!) because we want to buy a house and really need the extra money. Sara works part-time and takes two classes and watches Joe. Even though I didn't nurse her, she is very supportive and helpful. Honestly, I wish she had more freedom, and I think she could if I felt comfortable with other babysitters, which might happen if Joe wasn't nursing anymore. Also, I just feel like I am too tired to be creative, so I am having a hard time figuring out what to do if I am not nursing.

First/last nursing times to go: I am here when Joe wakes up, but only half of the time when he goes to bed. I think wake-up nursing will be hard to lose because we both love it, and I'll work on that last. Bedtime and nighttime may be first because he is used to me being gone sometimes, and Sara already has a routine. Then we could work on daytime.

How to include Joe: We tried to talk about weaning (real relaxed) with Joe, but he didn't seem to understand too much other than to pat my breasts and say he loves "Nee." I'm going to try to explain what we're doing, and remind him, and then see what he does. He already knows that older kids don't nurse anymore. He knows his cousin had a weaning party (at 18 months), and he wants one, though I don't think he totally gets that the party meant his cousin never nursed again. My friend at work has a kids' book about weaning that she said we could borrow. So, we'll read that. We're going full on with the new choices thing: a new sippy cup with water in it, a new night light for the room, and anything he can pick out himself. I hope that he'll feel like he got to be a part of things this way.

Plan

1. **Prep week.** A full week of talking about it, starting with us switching to Sara's routine instead of nursing for bedtime. He loves the Clifford calendar that his grandma gave him, so I am going to let him cross off days until "new bedtime."

2. **Then Sara takes care of bedtime, all the time at first.** I will go to the basement or run an errand so that Joe knows I am not there. Sara has a good routine: playtime, snack, books in bed, and then she sits in the rocking chair by the bed until Joe falls asleep. I am going to work into that routine. I'll start with doing snack and bath, and then, eventually, do it all. I think after two weeks of not nursing to sleep, he'll be used to it.

3. **Second: Nighttime.** I think it will be easy until he has some pain or other problem. Normally, the waking is so short and easy that I think I can give a drink instead, and sit in the rocker and sing to him. It is possible that he will cry, so I am going to prepare him for that during the first week. I am going to say that we both might be sad during the night, but that I will be there for him, and never leave him when he is sad. I'm going to encourage him to say what he thinks about it (he knows how to say several feelings). I think we may have a few bad nights with this, but will be okay after that. I am going to see if I can schedule work so that I am there in the middle of the night for at least three nights, even if I can't be for bedtime.

4. **After that, distractions during the day and naptime.** I will stand, not offer but won't refuse, will try distractions first with going outdoors, then with some new little toys and activities. I am going to

commit to getting through things without nursing. It may be hard at first, but I will be ready to do it. Trying to remember that I'm not abandoning him! I'll still be there—just not nursing. Naptime: decided we needed another routine, and I need exercise. Whichever of us is with him will take him for a walk; he loves that. He usually falls asleep in the stroller so we will let him nap like that while we get a walk in.

5. **Special situations.** I feel like there was a time when Joe couldn't have handled things without nursing but now, with so much experience of me being at work and having Sara comfort him, I really think he can handle it. I think I am the one who needs to be strong and commit. I am going to say the same thing each time: "We will have hugs and kisses and snuggles, and we will feel better soon." And I will just give him lots of love.

6. **Last first-morning nursing.** For now, I will not worry about this one. We need it after being away from each other. When it is time to work on it, I will get out of bed when Joe wakes up or, if I've been up all night, Sara will help. We will offer breakfast and play. Joe loves coconut milk, so we can offer that in the morning if he doesn't want to get out of bed. If I am desperately tired, and he really won't get up, I am giving myself permission to let him lie next to me and watch some PBS Kids on my phone. He'll probably think that is so cool that he'll forget about nursing.

7. **Goal.** I want Joe to be fully weaned by his 3rd birthday, and he can have a big kid/weaning party and make all the decisions about what he wants for the party. But I don't care if we are still nursing in the morning for longer. I think I'm okay with that.

Step Four: Implement and Evaluate

It can be easier both to implement and to evaluate with an older child than with a baby. If you have prepared your older child, and explained your plan and, hopefully, gotten some agreement from him, you should be able to begin putting your plans into practice quickly and easily. If this isn't the case, you might consider any difficulty you are having as a signal that something isn't working for you, your child, or your plan.

Try to stick with each step of your plan as you get to it for a while. There really is no other way to find out what works for you and what doesn't, because most changes take at least a few repetitions before they stick. Even when a child is upset, you can stick with your plan as long as you are physically there for them, comforting them, and explaining (very simply) if needed, though some children are *more* upset with constant explanations, so observe carefully. You can remind them by using stock phrases ("We're not nursing at night but I will be with you while you fall back to sleep. Would you like a back rub or a story?" etc.). Make sure you accept all emotions that your child expresses. They are all normal, and expressing them is how most of us process and move past them. At first, you may not get much more than anger or tears in response to anything you do. Within a few days, you should be getting calmer responses, even if your child still isn't thrilled about the change.

If you've been consistent, and are still getting a lot of anger or tears after quite a few tries, it may be time to consider revamping your plan. Talk with your child and see if you can understand what is bothering them. Often, we assume we know what it is (not nursing), when it is really something else. Sometimes, the words we use are upsetting to kids, and we don't realize it. My older son really hated when I mentioned phrases, such as "big kid" or "big boy," and it took me a while to get that he knew what I didn't: that I used that language when I wanted him to do something he wasn't ready for. Sometimes, it is the tone we use, or the substitutes we give, that upset kids. Perhaps you've been offering that backrub to your child because they have always loved them, but they don't want backrubs to be used as a substitute. You could ask them what would be a better option and give several choices.

If things don't resolve after some further planning and implementation, it may be time to take a break and regroup. Did you allow your child to be invested in your weaning plan by making choices and agreeing to the steps as you took them? Is he feeling a sense of loss that you can help him talk through and process? Are there things in your life that are causing stress for you or your child? Are there difficult feelings between you and your child that have traditionally only been calmed and sweetened by nursing? Are you giving him lots of focused time with you other than nursing? Is he scared of anything? Is it possible that your child just isn't quite ready yet, and is it possible to give him just a bit more time? Often, things that don't work now, work well just a few weeks or months down the line.

If you need to take a break from your plan, and worry that it will ruin all of your hard weaning work, just remember that communication is the key. You can explain to your child that the weaning plan is making everyone sad. You can tell him that you want to "pause" and think about how much you love each other and how to do things better. You can look at other techniques, and discuss them with him to see if there is anything that will be acceptable to both of you while you figure things out. For example, some moms who have paused have agreed with their child to nurse again before bed, but only if they ended the feeding a little earlier than they normally would (see techniques for this in Chapter 8 of this book), and then followed a bedtime routine. Don't forget to ask your child for his ideas for solutions. Kids can really surprise us with their practical wisdom.

Continue to work with your child. You are setting up a framework of communication, respect, and love that will last a lifetime, even as *this* stage, I promise, will not! Breathe, assess, and be flexible. Seriously, despite the jokes people make about how their kid would nurse forever if allowed, even families whose weanings are completely unscheduled and child-led still wean, and often a lot earlier than their parents think they will. You are on the road to weaning, even if you're driving slowly.

So how did Joe's weaning plan go?

His mom says, "Great! Every time we made a change, we talked about it and got used to the idea for a while. Then when we did it, he usually cried the first time or two but, with lots of comfort and reassurance, he got it. He nursed for the last time the morning of his 3rd birthday/weaning party. I thought he might ask again the next morning, but he didn't."

Another Mother's Story of Weaning a Child Older Than 2

Janine K.

Daughter #1 nursed for 18 months while I struggled with milk supply. In hindsight, it was probably due to her sleeping long stretches at night, which, for a working mom, might be seen as a benefit, but can be a detriment for milk supply.

I nursed her daily at lunchtime, but keeping up with bottles at daycare became a struggle because she loved bottles and sippy cups. At about 14 months, she asked for milk one morning when she woke up, so I proceeded to snuggle with her in bed and offered the breast. She said "No, milk!" and signed it repeatedly. She wanted a sippy cup of cow's milk! I knew at that moment that our nursing relationship might be coming to an end. Had I offered her cow's milk too soon? Did she like the independence of the sippy cup? Should we have co-slept? Should I have used a sling or wrap?

Weaning was a fairly quick process. She continued to nurse before bed for a few more months, but she didn't fall asleep at the breast. She became fussier at bedtime. My husband became the bedtime guru and could snuggle with her to fall asleep, so it was a team effort: Mommy to nurse, Daddy to snuggle to sleep. If she woke in the night, we would both try to do what we did best (nurse and/or snuggle), until one of them worked and ultimately, the snuggles were most desired.

I became pregnant with daughter #2 when she was almost

completely weaned. Once my belly started to get in the way, snuggling with Daddy was more common and, when #2 came along, Daddy was most responsible for bedtime comfort while I tended to the baby.

Daughter #2 nursed for 3.5 years, and I kept up my milk production more successfully than with #1. I believe this was because she slept more frequently in our bed, I had the support of La Leche League mothers, she woke more frequently at night, and she didn't eat as much during the day. I nursed at lunchtime, as I did with #1, but unlike #1, #2 didn't like bottles as much. She'd rather wait for me to nurse. We nursed frequently throughout the evening and at night. When she was in her own bed at about age 2, we'd nurse to sleep in her bed and she'd fall asleep. She'd usually make her way to my bed at some point, where she'd nurse and sleep the rest of the night.

When she was almost 3, we started talking about turning 3, and not needing my milk anymore. At night, we'd listen to music, and I'd say that she could have three songs. Then she'd ask for another and another, and she'd nurse while both of us fell asleep. Slowly, we were able to stop nursing after three songs, then two songs, then one song. At this point, I don't think I had much milk. I'd continue to ask her if anything was coming out, to which she'd reply "yes, and it tastes like vanilla ice cream" (still her favorite ice cream flavor). Weaning was a gradual, fun, and memorable process. I remember it more clearly than with #1, maybe because it lasted longer, maybe because it wasn't so sudden, maybe because she was the focus, or maybe because I was more experienced and knowledgeable so that I could maintain the relationship longer, and with more compassion.

To other breastfeeding parents I would say "cherish every moment." While you may want breastfeeding to end so you can sleep, or have your body back, or have more independence, these things don't really change. Your non-nursing toddler and preschooler will still need you to put them to bed, and be there for them when they wake up in the middle of the night. Instead of nursing, you will be rocking, reading, telling stories, singing, etc. So, enjoy it for as long as you can, as it's probably easier than the alternative, at least until the baby decides the nursing need has been met, and weaning gradually happens.

I feel like compassion = patience. I can admit that I was less patient with my 1st, and likely less compassionate. When she didn't fall asleep nursing, I wasn't sure what else to do! I am grateful for my husband's support, and patience, and his ability to comfort her to sleep.

Child-Led Plans, Partial Weaning, and Abrupt Weaning

CHAPTER 10

Child-Led Plans

This may sound counterintuitive, but if weaning is a spectrum, even moms who are willing for it to be child-led, and have no end-date in mind, may still need to have some plan for how to handle certain situations. Many mothers in the U.S. no longer feel comfortable nursing in public after their children reach a certain age, and they need to think about how to work on this with their children. Other mothers find that they don't like to discuss their continued nursing with others, and have to figure out how to explain this to their children without making it sound like a shameful practice that must be hidden.

Breastfeeding will end for those on the child-led end of the spectrum too. You may find yourself wanting to change a few things as you go along, even while you plan to continue as long as needed. For example, some mothers find themselves needing more sleep than they thought they would as their child gets older, and find that they want to curb breastfeeding at certain times, without planning to wean entirely. This is usually called partial weaning, and is discussed in the next section.

149

A Mother's Story of Child-led Weaning

Kat P.

Just as every birth story has its own unique twists and turns, so does every weaning story. I was blessed to have the opportunity to allow my daughter to stop breastfeeding when she wanted to, and to follow her lead in the process. I would say that weaning began the first time she had a taste of solid food at 6 months (though her primary source of nutrition was still breast milk throughout the first year), and lasted through her last nursing, at about 27 months, and even for a few months beyond that, when we would both revisit the idea of nursing, and what it had meant for us.

My daughter's weaning was gradual. At about 15 months, I remember wanting to drop one common nursing time for her—the 5 a.m. feeding—feeling she could make it to sun-up just fine without it. So, my husband went in to soothe her at that time for a couple of weeks. This is the only one I remember pushing for. Other than that, the frequency just seemed to slowly melt away. I liked using the "don't offer, don't refuse" strategy around age 2 to test the waters. In the end, I would have willingly nursed her further into the future. I never got to a point where it bothered me. But in the last few weeks, it was clear that she had filled that need, and at every nursing I wondered, "Is this the last one?" I had time along the way to contemplate it all, which really contributed to how smoothly it went. Acknowledging that she had fully weaned was a bit sad for me, but I knew deeply that our nursing relationship had been very positive and beneficial for both of us, and that it had ended naturally and at the right time for us.

Once or twice, many weeks later, my daughter asked to nurse. I let her try, and she would just touch her lips to my breast for a quick second and then move on. It was like a new swimmer touching the side of the pool to make sure it is still there. About a year after she had weaned completely, she saw me naked out of the shower and said, "I want milk from your body." I explained that there probably wasn't any left, but that if she wanted to try, she could. She didn't want to, but was a bit sad. I just gave her a big hug and said that what we had when we nursed was great, but now we have lots of other ways to show love. That was a really special moment for me as a mother—tinged with happiness, sadness, laughter, and pride all at once.

Now that she is 4, she looks forward to seeing friends from our mom-to-mom group, occasionally "nurses" one of her dolls, and speaks excitedly about having babies someday and giving them "mama's milk." These are the kinds of benefits of breastfeeding that no medical study can show: just a healthy way of looking at our bodies, nature, and our place in it all as women.

Partial Weaning

When families decide to set aside blocks of times during which the child will no longer nurse, for whatever reason, it is usually called "partial weaning," though it can also be called, "night weaning" or "day weaning." Partial weaning isn't usually recommended for children under the age of 1 (and sometimes isn't healthy for some children even after that) because younger babies and children truly have caloric, sucking, and reconnection needs that cannot easily be met in other ways.

Partial weaning, like all weaning, consists of dropping nursing sessions, whether completely or gradually. However, unlike general weaning, you will probably be doing this with several sessions, deferring all of them until a specific time (bedtime, when the sun comes up, whatever you have chosen). If you are partially weaning a child under the age of 1, there is a good chance that your milk supply will be affected by dropping several sessions at once. Additionally, your child will need supplementation if she is hungry when you are not nursing her, and she will still have a strong need for your presence.

Note: Even with older nurslings, moms may see their supplies dip a bit as they cut nursing sessions.

Before you partially wean, make sure to take some time to observe the situation as objectively as you can to see where your desire to make this change originates from, and whether partial weaning will address the issue. Also, observe whether your child seems to be ready for a change. Children naturally sleep differently than adults for developmental reasons, and most parents find that their nighttime parenting job continues in some fashion, even after night weaning. If you are considering night weaning, plan for how you will compassionately meet nighttime needs when you are not nursing, whatever the age of your child.

A partial weaning during the day may look very much like any other weaning and many of the tips in the Practical Advice from Moms section in Chapter 8 of this book will be helpful. But when night weaning, parents will probably find distractions too disruptive, focusing instead on alternative methods of comforting and putting children back to sleep, so some of the usual tips may not apply.

Here are some of the more useful tips for partial weaning. Remember that changes may take several repetitions to work.

❋ Allow Your Child to Make Choices.

This is one of the best ways to include your child in weaning plans. Make sure that the options you provide her are all acceptable, and that you are willing to abide by her choices. Perhaps she can choose which cup to drink water from during the night, or whether she wants a song or some patting to go back to sleep. Maybe she decides which activity will replace nursing sessions during day weaning.

❋ "Tank-Up."

If you are night weaning, make sure bedtime nursing provides a full meal so that your child can make it until you have chosen to nurse again. Using breast compression and massage as you nurse can help make sure that this meal is satisfying enough to last awhile.

● Keep Expectations Clear and Remind Kids of Them.

Simple words, clear expectations, and gentle reminders will keep all of you on track. Most kids need reminders and preparation *before* problems arise to be successful.

● Don't Encourage More Milk Production When Actively Weaning.

If you feel uncomfortably full during partial weaning, you can pump just until you feel better (stopping here rather than fully draining your breasts), so that your body gets the message to make less.

● Stock Phrases and Clear Statements.

It is helpful if everyone in the family is using the same simple language while weaning. See what feels good to you, and try to stick to it so your child isn't confused. Make sure you are stating clearly what you *want* your child to do, not just telling her what *not* to do. For example, when you must say "no" to a nursing session, how will you do it? Rather than trying to explain every situation, it can be useful to say the same basic thing every day, such as, "We will nurse at bedtime. Let's go play_____." (if weaning during the day). You can edit as needed, but you will want to keep the first part of it the same, most likely. It reminds your child of the plan. The second part tells her what you *will* do. Notice that the word "no" doesn't even need to be used. If weaning at night, the stock phrase might be something like, "We will nurse when the sun comes up. Do you want a drink of water?"

● Keep in Mind What Is Developmental Normal for Your Child.

Breastfeeding and gentle-parenting experts know that sleep, interest in solids, independence, and other things are developmental stages that children move into when they are ready. Expect age-appropriate reactions, abilities, and behaviors from your child.

* **Acknowledge Your Child's Feelings.**

Even if you don't understand them, their feelings are legitimate and you can accept them, help name them if they need you to, and help process them. This is another great parenting skill that will serve you for a long time to come.

Note: If you need information specific to weaning from the pump during working hours, please see the Frequently Asked Question about pumping in Chapter 7.

A Mother's Story of Partial Weaning

L.S.

If you would have told me I'd be nursing a 2-year-old, I would never have believed you! I was just trying to do at least a year, but then when my son turned 1-year-old, he still seemed like such a baby, and I couldn't imagine stopping. He loved nursing, and I mostly loved it too.

When my son was almost 2, I found myself frustrated with daytime nursing more than nighttime. He slept in my bed, and usually slept well. He would wake a few times, but just sucked for a minute, and then fell asleep again. I quit my job when he was 2 months old (before my maternity leave even ended), so we were home together all the time during the day. That had been great originally, but now it felt like we were nursing all the time, anytime I sat down, or we had a break from activity. He ate lots of solid foods, but that didn't seem to dampen his desire to nurse at all. But it did make me think he could probably get by without nursing.

My partner and I decided to wean him just during the day. He could nurse when he woke in the morning (he wasn't napping anymore), and when he went to bed, and during the night. We talked about it a lot, preparing him for a couple of weeks. But when we came to it, it was a fight! I was unprepared for that, and wasn't sure how to handle it. When I said no to him, he would hit me, and scream and cry. I talked with

154

some other moms who said to just stay strong, acknowledge his feelings, and repeat that we would nurse at bedtime. I tried to do more fun things, and find other ways to stop him from nursing than saying "no." That helped. I tried to keep things to do, and snacks at hand all the time so that he was distracted, and if he asked directly, I just said "Nursing will be at bedtime," and quickly found something to do. If he tried to hit me, I held him, and snuggled, and played his favorite tickle game. I don't know if that was the right thing, but it worked. It took us about a week, though he sometimes asks, even now. He doesn't seem to expect it, though. Just likes to ask.

We night weaned a year later. We talked with him about it, and then, at night, just told him "Nursing will be in the morning." I stuck with it, even when he cried, snuggling and patting him, and saying "Mama loves you. I'm here" (my partner came up with that part). Again, it took about a week. He is 3 and a half now, and only nurses at bedtime.

Abrupt Weaning

Life can change in unexpected and unfortunate ways, and parents can find themselves in situations that require heartbreaking decisions. As a loving parent in a situation beyond your control, you want to know how to be as compassionate as possible in such circumstances, and I can assure you that your child will benefit from your consideration. Your situation is probably difficult enough, and you will want to avoid any impacts on your body, your child, and your connection, which could further complicate your lives.

An abrupt weaning may mean that there is no tapering of breastfeeding at all: the baby was nursing yesterday and isn't today. It may also mean a few days of removing nursing sessions until they are gone. Closely observe your body and your child as you go through the process of an abrupt weaning.

For mother's transition, experts and moms recommend:

* When you feel full, pump or hand express only until you feel comfortable, and don't drain the breast. This will lower the "demand" side of supply and demand to give your body the message to make less.

* Cold cabbage leaves (or other cold compresses) in the bra can help relieve engorgement.

* Wear a firm bra for support (one size larger than usual so it does not get too tight).

* Reduce your salt intake, but not your fluids.

* Be aware that you might experience grief and other difficult emotions as you wean abruptly and get support, if needed (Mohrbacher & Kendall-Tackett, 2010).

* Massage with warmth to help prevent blockages.

* Add foods to your diet that depress supply and minimize foods that boost it. For example, sage, mint, parsley (among others) can lower supply while oats, alfalfa, barley, and sesame seeds (among others) can boost supply. The book *Mother Food* by Hilary Jacobson can be very helpful in identifying these.

For a child's transition, experts and moms recommend:

* Be prepared with other healthy foods and milk substitutes, if necessary, so that the child's nutrition and health is not compromised.

* Be present, physically and emotionally, as much as possible. Weaning can be stressful in addition to the original event that is causing abrupt weaning. Experts say that children who have positive emotional supports during stress have much better outcomes than those who don't (Center on the Developing Child, 2007; Mohrbacher & Kendall-Tackett, 2010).

Final Thoughts

You are on the weaning journey. As you travel, the love you show is a beacon of joy and safety for your child. The time and care that you are putting in, and the loving partnership you are creating, show your child that she is valuable and that her needs matter. What a priceless gift you are giving. This gift will endure, and its impact will grow as you watch your teenager, and then adult child, move into the world with confidence and independence and, most importantly, a sense of compassion for others.

Take your time and enjoy the weaning process, if circumstances allow. The day will come sooner than you can imagine when your job is mostly done, and you'll miss these days of tiny warm bodies and physical closeness. Trust your instincts as a parent, your child, and your bond. You're moving forward, together.

References

American Academy of Pediatrics. (2017). *Starting solid foods*. Retrieved from: https://healthychildren.org/English/ages-stages/baby/feeding-nutrition/Pages/Switching-To-Solid-Foods.aspx

American Academy of Pediatric Dentistry. (2015). *Policy on the use of xylitol*. Retrieved from: http://www.aapd.org/media/Policies_Guidelines/P_Xylitoll.pdf

Australian Breastfeeding Association. (2013). *Continuing breastfeeding after separation and divorce*. Retrieved from: https://www.breastfeeding.asn.au/bf-info/breastfeeding-and-law/continuing-breastfeeding-after-separation-and-divorce?q=bf-info%2Fbreastfeeding-and-law%2Fcontinuing-breastfeeding-after-separation-and-divorce

Bengson, D. (1999). *How weaning happens*. Schaumburg, IL: La Leche League International.

Berkowitz, R.J. (2006). Mutans streptococci: Acquisition and transmission. *Pediatric Dentistry, 28*(2). Retrieved from: http://www.aapd.org/assets/1/25/Berkowitz-28-2.pdf

Centers for Disease Control and Prevention. (2007). Does breastfeeding reduce the risk of pediatric overweight? *CDC: Division of Nutrition and Physical Activity: Research to Practice Series No. 4*. Retrieved from: https://www.cdc.gov/nccdphp/dnpa/nutrition/pdf/breastfeeding_r2p.pdf

Center on the Developing Child. (2007). *InBrief: The impact of early adversity on children's development*. Retrieved from: http://developingchild.harvard.edu/resources/inbrief-the-impact-of-early-adversity-on-childrens-development/

Coloroso, B. (2012). *Parenting through crisis: Helping kids in times of loss, grief, and change* (International ed.). Toronto, ON: Penguin.

Eidelman, A. I., & Schandler, R.J. (2012). Breastfeeding and the use of human milk. *Pediatrics, 129*(3). doi:10.1542/peds.2011-3552

Erickson, P.R., & Mazhari, E. (1999). Investigation of the role of human breast milk in caries development. *Pediatric Dentistry, 21*, 2.

Faber, A., & Mazlish, E. (2012). *How to talk so kids will listen & listen so kids will talk* (updated ed.). New York: Scribner Classics.

Fleischer, D. M., Sicherer, S., Greenhawt, M., Campbell, D., Chan, E. S., Muraro, A., Halken, S., Katz, Y., Ebisawa, M., Eichenfield, L., & Sampson, H. (2015). Consensus communication on early peanut introduction and the prevention of peanut allergy in high-risk infants. *World Allergy Organization Journal, 8*(1). doi:10.1186/s40413-015-0076-x

Flower, H. (2003). *Adventures in tandem nursing: Breastfeeding during pregnancy and beyond.* Schaumburg, IL: La Leche League International.

Flower, H. (2005). *Adventures in gentle discipline: A parent-to-parent guide.* Schaumburg, IL: La Leche League International.

Forssten, S. D., Björklund, M., & Ouwehand, A. C. (2010). *Streptococcus mutans, caries and simulation models. Nutrients, 2*(3), 290–298. doi:http://doi.org/10.3390/nu2030290

Gonzalez, C. (2012). *My child won't eat!: How to enjoy mealtimes without worry* (2nd ed.). London: Printer and Martin, LTD.

Hale, T. W., & Rowe, H. E. (2017). *Medications & mothers' milk* (17th ed.). New York: Springer Publishing Company, LLC.

Higham, B. (2017, March 20). Sleep like a baby. *Women's Health Today Blog.* Retrieved from: https://womenshealthtoday.blog/2017/03/14/sleep-like-a-baby/

Huggins, K., & Ziedrich, L. (2007). *The nursing mothers guide to weaning: How to bring breastfeeding to a gentle close, and how to decide when the time is right* (Revised ed.). Boston, MA: Harvard Common Press.

Humphrey, S. (2003). *The nursing mother's herbal* (Human Body Library). Minneapolis, MN: Fairview Press.

Iida, H., Auinger, P., Billings, R.J., & Weitzman, M. (2007). Association between infant breastfeeding and early childhood caries in the United States. *Pediatrics, 120,* 4. Retrieved from: http://pediatrics.aappublications.org/content/120/4/e944?sso=1&sso_redirect_count=1&nfstatus=401&nftoken=00000000-0000-0000-0000-000000000000&nfstatusdescription=ERROR%3a+No+local+token

Institute for Reproductive Health. (2017). *Lactational Amenorrhea Method (LAM).* Retrieved from: http://irh.org/lam/

Jacobson, H. (2016). *Healing breastfeeding grief: How mothers feel and heal when breastfeeding does not go as hoped.* Ashland, OR: Rosalind Press.

Jacobson, H. (2007). *Mother food: A breastfeeding diet guide with lactogenic foods and herbs.* Ashland, OR: Rosalind Press.

Kendall-Tackett, K. A. (2017). *Depression in new mothers: Causes, consequences, and treatment alternatives, 3rd Ed.* London and New York: Routledge, Taylor, & Francis Group.

Kurcinka, M. S. (2000). *Kids, parents, and power struggles: Winning for a lifetime.* New York: HarperCollins.

La Leche League, International. (2016). *When should my baby start solids?* Retrieved from: http://www.llli.org/faq/solids.html

Lönnerdal, B. (2013), Bioactive proteins in breast milk. *Journal of Paediatric & Child Health, 49*, 1-7. doi:10.1111/jpc.12104

Mayo Clinic Staff. (2015). *Extended breast-feeding: What you need to know.* Retrieved from: http://www.mayoclinic.org/healthy-lifestyle/infant-and-toddler-health/in-depth/extended-breastfeeding/art-20046962

Mohebbi, S. Z., Virtanen, J. I., Vahid-Golpayegani, M., & Vehkalahti, M. M. (2008). Feeding habits as determinants of early childhood caries in a population where prolonged breastfeeding is the norm. *Community Dentistry and Oral Epidemiology, 36*(4), 363-369. doi:10.1111/j.1600-0528.2007.00408.x

Mohrbacher, N. (2010). *Breastfeeding answers made simple: A guide for helping mothers.* Amarillo, TX: Hale Publishing.

Mohrbacher, N. (2012). Do older babies need night feedings? *Breastfeeding Reporter Blog.* Retrieved from http://www.nancymohrbacher.com/articles/2012/10/31/do-older-babies-need-night-feedings.html

Mohrbacher, N. (2014a). *Working and breastfeeding made simple.* Amarillo, TX: Praeclarus Press.

Mohrbacher, N. (2014b). *Infographic on breast storage capacity.* Breastfeeding Reporter Blog. Retrieved from: http://www.nancymohrbacher.com/articles/2014/1/17/infographic-on-breast-storage-capacity.html

Mohrbacher, N., & Kendall-Tackett, K. (2010). *Breastfeeding made simple: Seven natural laws for nursing mothers.* Oakland, CA: New Harbinger.

Montgomery, A., Dermer, A., Eglash, A., Quiogue, M., Saenz, R., & Tobolic, T.J. (2014). *Breastfeeding, Family Physicians supporting.* Retrieved from: http://www.aafp.org/about/policies/all/breastfeeding-support.html

Murtagh, L., & Moulton, A. D. (2011). *Working mothers, breastfeeding, and the law.* Retrieved from: https://www.ncbi.nlm.nih.gov/pmc/articles/PMC3020209/

Newman, J., & Kernerman, E. (2009). *Breastfeed a toddler - Why on earth?* Retrieved from: https://www.breastfeedinginc.ca/informations/breastfeed-a-toddler-why-on-earth/

Ockwell-Smith, S. (2014). *Self-settling – What really happens when you teach a baby to self soothe to sleep.* Retrieved from: https://sarahockwell-smith.com/2014/06/30/self-settling-what-really-happens-when-you-teach-a-baby-to-self-soothe-to-sleep/

Ockwell-Smith, S. (2015). *The gentle sleep book: A guide for calm babies, toddlers and pre-schoolers.* London: Piatkus.

Oddy, W. H., Kendall, G. E., Li, J., Jacoby, P., Robinson, M., Klerk, N. H., Silburn, S. R., Zubrick S. R., Landau, L.I., & Stanley, F.J. (2009). The long-term effects of breastfeeding on child and adolescent mental health: A pregnancy cohort study followed for 14 years. *Journal of Pediatrics, 156*(4), 568-574. doi:10.1016/j.jpeds.2009.10.020

Pantley, E. (2005). *The no-cry sleep solution: Gentle ways to help your baby sleep through the night*. Chicago, IL: McGraw-Hill.

Peretz, B., Ram D., Odont, E.A., & Efrat, Y. (2003). Preschool caries as an indicator of future caries: A longitudinal study. *Pediatric Dentistry 25*, 2. Retrieved from: http://www.aapd.org/assets/1/25/Peretz2-03.pdf

Pryor, G., & Huggins, K. (2007). *Nursing mother, working mother: The essential guide to breastfeeding your baby before and after you return to work* (Revised ed.). Boston, MA: Harvard Common Press.

Roche-Paull, R. (2010). *Breastfeeding in combat boots: A survival guide to successful breastfeeding while serving in the military*. Amarillo, TX: Hale Publishing.

Rosenberg, M.B. (2003). *Nonviolent communication: A language of life*. Encinitas, CA: PuddleDancer Press.

Rugg-Gunn, A. J., Roberts, G. J., & Wright, W. G. (1985). Effect of human milk on plaque pH in situ and enamel dissolution in vitro compared with bovine milk, lactose, and sucrose. *Caries Research, 19*(4), 327-334.

Sears, W. (n.d.). *Weaning*. Retrieved from: http://www.askdrsears.com/topics/feeding-eating/breastfeeding/faqs/weaning

Sears, W., Sears, M., Sears, R., & Sears, J. (2005). *The baby sleep book: The complete guide to a good night's rest for the whole family*. Sears Parenting Library. New York: Hatchette Book Group.

Siegel, D. J., & Bryson, T. P. (2014). *No-drama discipline: The whole-brain way to calm the chaos and nurture your child's developing mind*. New York: Bantam Books.

Slevin, A. (2007). *Breastfeeding with postpartum depression*. Retrieved from: http://nurse-practitioners-and-physician-assistants.advanceweb.com/Article/Breastfeeding-with-Postpartum-Depression.aspx

Stuart-Macadam, P., & Dettwyler, K. A. (1995). *Breastfeeding: Biocultural perspectives*. New York: Aldine De Gruyter.

Walters, S. (2008). Breastfeeding during pregnancy. *New Beginnings, 25*(1), 32-33.

Weschler, T. (2015). *Taking charge of your fertility, 20th anniversary edition: The definitive guide to natural birth control, pregnancy achievement, and reproductive health*. New York: William Morrow.

World Health Organization. (2017). *The World Health Organization's infant feeding recommendation*. Retrieved from: http://www.who.int/nutrition/topics/infantfeeding_recommendation/en/

Wiessinger, D., West, D., & Pitman, T. (2010). *The womanly art of breastfeeding: Completely revised and updated 8th edition*. New York: Ballantine Books.

Wiessinger, D., West, D., Smith, L. J., & Pitman, T. (2014). *Sweet sleep: Nighttime and naptime strategies for the breastfeeding family.* New York: Ballantine Books.

Winstein, M. (1997). *Your fertility signals: Using them to achieve or avoid pregnancy naturally.* St. Louis, MO: Smooth Stone Press.

About the Author

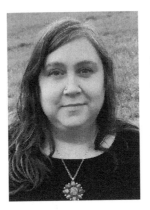

Winema Wilson Lanoue has been working with breastfeeding families since 2002, providing support and information throughout the entire breastfeeding journey. She promotes breastfeeding and loving parenting through this work and through her writing, always striving to empower and encourage parents.

A mother, herself, Winema truly believes that gentle parenting is the key to a healthy society. Aside from writing and editing works about parenting, Winema is a gluten free baker and crafter of stories, songs and other art. She works to create a home and a life full of love, fun, and compassion.

You can follow and/or contact Winema Wilson Lanoue at:
WinemaWilsonLanoue.com
https://www.facebook.com/winemawilsonlanoue/
https://twitter.com/WinemaLanoue

Photo by Sally Butler Provo, 2017

Made in the USA
Middletown, DE
12 March 2018